BY THE EDITORS OF

CONSUMER GUIDE®

EMERGENCY FIRST AID for CATS

This publication is not to be used in place of a veterinarian, but merely to guide you in helping the injured animal until you can get professional care. Our guidelines are based on what will happen with most cats in most situations. However, there are always a few exceptions where the cat may not respond to your first aid as expected; these cats will need professional care even sooner.

Manufactured in the United States of America

About the Author: Sheldon Rubin, DVM, is a practicing veterinarian in Chicago, Il. He received his Doctorate of Veterinary Medicine from the University of Illinois in 1968. Dr. Rubin has served as President and as Secretary of the Chicago Veterinary Medical Association and is also a member of several state and national associations dealing with the practice of veterinary medicine.

Cover Photo: Caravaglia/International Stock Photo
Illustrations: Mike Muir

Contents

Contents

Dealing with an Emergency

Have you ever seen a cat injured in a fight or hit by a car? Perhaps you could only shake your head and walk away. Not because you didn't care, but because you didn't know how to approach and examine the animal, or what to do next. Especially if you have a cat of your own, you'll want to be prepared, for your pet depends on you for help in an emergency situation.

If we, like Dr. Doolittle, could "talk with the animals" it would be easy to find out what they'd gotten into, and where it hurt. Since we can't, in order to apply the proper treatment we must be able to identify signs that pinpoint the problem. The First Aid section of this book lists the most common emergencies alphabetically. When the nature of an injury or condition is not readily apparent, signs are listed at the beginning of the section to help you identify the problem.

The purpose of first aid is to relieve suffering and stabilize your cat's vital signs until professional help is obtained. This book will give you the information and techniques you'll need to confidently administer first aid, and perhaps save the life of a pet. Clear directions are listed step-by-step. Where more than one procedure is necessary to perform a step, each specific action is described in substeps a, b, c, etc. An example of this occurs in Step 6 of Shock. The directions are further clarified with graphic illustrations.

The "why" of these procedures is explained in the back of the book. This section also includes preventive measures that can eliminate or minimize some hazards that could be dangerous to your pet.

The index is cross-referenced to make it easy to find the page you need. Many emergency conditions will be found under several headings. For example: "Snakebite" will also be listed under "Bite, poisonous snake," "Bite, nonpoisonous snake," "Poisonous snakebite," and "Nonpoisonous snakebite."

Because minutes count in an emergency situation, you'll want to have a first aid kit prepared. It needn't be elaborate; suggested items are listed on page 158. Keep the kit and this book together in a convenient place, and take both with you when you travel with your cat.

We suggest you take the time to thoroughly familiarize yourself with the contents of this book. Certain sections are especially important. When a cat is choking or unconscious, speed is vital if the cat is to live. Therefore, it is of primary importance that you know how to give artificial respiration and CPR (cardiopulmonary resuscitation). It will also be most helpful if you know exactly how to approach and restrain a cat if an accident does occur. The method of restraint that you choose will depend largely upon whether the cat is cooperative or uncooperative. It may become necessary for you to protect your own self from injury caused by an uncooperative cat's five weapons—its mouth and four sets of claws.

In addition to the information you'll need to contact your own veterinarian, there is a line below to list the phone number of the Poison Control Center in your area. You will find them very helpful should it become necessary to contact them. The number is in your phone book.

EMERGENCY INFORMATION

VETERINARIAN'S NAME: _____

EMERGENCY PHONE: _____

HOSPITAL PHONE: _____

HOSPITAL ADDRESS: _____

POISON CONTROL CENTER PHONE: _____

Approaching an Injured Cat

STEP 1: Approach slowly, speaking in a reassuring tone of voice.

STEP 2: Move close to the cat without touching it.

STEP 3: Stoop down to the cat. While continuing to speak, observe its eyes and body language.

a. If the cat is wide-eyed, ears back, growling and hissing, DO NOT attempt to pet it. Proceed to RESTRAINING AN UNCOOPERATIVE CAT, page 13.

b. If the cat is shivering and crouching, attempt to reassure it by petting, first behind the head. If this is permitted, pet the rest of the head and neck. Scratching the ears and stroking under the chin is often comforting. Proceed to RESTRAINING A COOPERATIVE CAT, page 8.

> **CAUTION:** A cat has five weapons: the mouth and four paws.

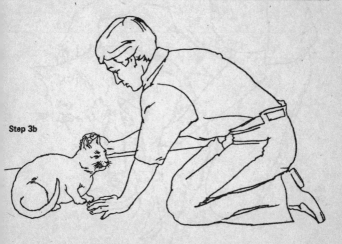

Step 3b

Restraining a Cooperative Cat

CAUTION: A cat has five weapons: the mouth and four paws.

A. If you have an assistant

STEP 1: Place the cat in your arms or lap or on a table or other raised surface using one of the three following methods:

Method 1

a. Position yourself so the cat's head is to your left.

b. Reach with your right hand over the cat's body and under its chest so the chest is resting in your palm.

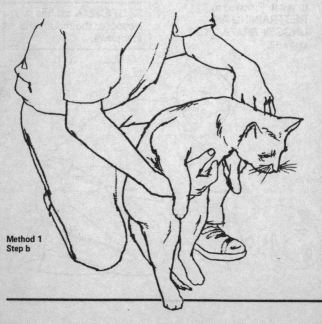

Method 1
Step b

c. Lift the cat firmly toward you so that its body is secured between your forearm and your body.

d. Grasp the top of the front legs with the fingers of your right hand, which is still supporting the chest.

e. Using the other hand, prevent the head from moving by grasping under the throat. Scratching the ears with this hand from under the throat is often very comforting.

f. Treatment can then be administered by your assistant while the cat is in your arms.

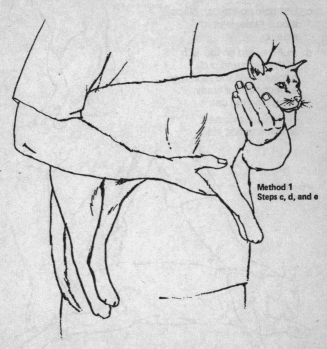

Method 1
Steps c, d, and e

continued

Method 2

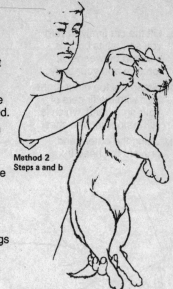

a. Grasp the loose skin on the back of the neck just below the ears. Lift the cat; most cats will become very submissive when this method is used.

b. Grasp the hind legs with your other hand to prevent scratching.

**Method 2
Steps a and b**

c. Still holding the cat, place it on a table, injured side up.

d. Pull forward on the skin of the neck and pull backward on the hind legs as if gently but firmly stretching the cat.

e. Have your assistant administer first aid.

**Method 2
Steps c and d**

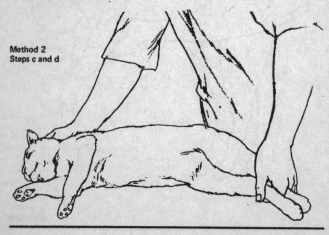

Method 3

a. Lift the cat by holding the loose skin on the back of the neck in one hand and the loose skin of the back in the other.

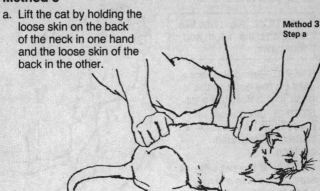

Method 3
Step a

b. Place the cat on a table or other raised surface and push the cat down firmly; it will be unable to use its claws.

c. Have your assistant administer first aid.

Method 3
Step b

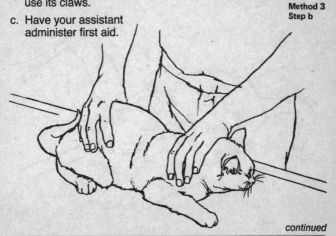

continued

B. If you are alone

> CAUTION: A cat has five
> weapons: the mouth and
> four paws.

STEP 1: Grasp the loose
skin on the back of the
neck just below the ears.

STEP 2: Lift the cat and
place it on its chest on a
table or other raised
surface.

STEP 3: If the cat will not
stay, place it in a large,
open box.

STEP 4: Administer
first aid.

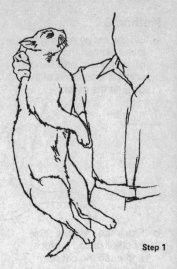

Step 1

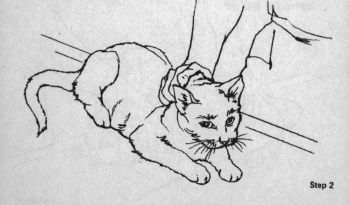

Step 2

Restraining an Uncooperative Cat

A. If you have an assistant

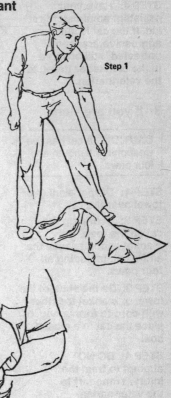

> CAUTION: A cat has five weapons: the mouth and four paws.

STEP 1: Drop a blanket or towel over the cat.

STEP 2: Scoop up the cat so the towel or blanket encompasses the entire cat, including all four paws.

Step 1

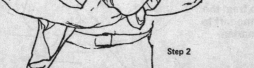

Step 2

continued

STEP 3: Expose only the injured area, keeping the rest of the cat covered.

STEP 4: Have your assistant administer first aid. If the cat is still very aggressive, transport untreated, still covered in the blanket or towel, to the veterinarian.

B. If you are alone

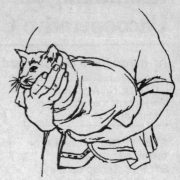

Step 3 Expose only the injured area; in this case, the cat has a head injury.

CAUTION: A cat has five weapons: the mouth and four paws.

STEP 1: Drop a blanket or towel over the cat.

STEP 2: Scoop up the cat so the towel or blanket encompasses the entire cat, including all four paws.

STEP 3: Tie the ends of the towel or blanket together with cord to form a bag, or place the cat in a closed box.

STEP 4: DO NOT attempt to treat the injury. Transport to the veterinarian.

Step 2

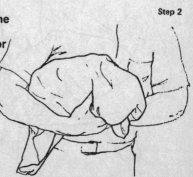

Transporting an Injured Cat

A. If the cat can be lifted

STEP 1: If the cat is cooperative:

a. Position yourself so the cat's head is to your left.

b. Reach with your right hand over the cat's body and under its chest so the chest is resting in your palm.

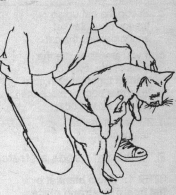

c. Lift the cat firmly toward you so that its body is secured between your forearm and your body.

d. Grasp the top of the front legs with the fingers of your right hand, which is still supporting the chest.

Step 1b

e. Using the other hand, prevent the head from moving by grasping under the throat. Scratching the ears with this hand from under the throat is often very comforting.

f. Transport to the veterinarian.

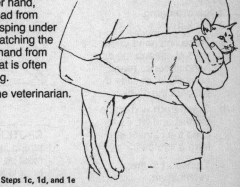

Steps 1c, 1d, and 1e

continued

STEP 2: If the cat is uncooperative:

a. Drop a blanket or towel over the cat.

b. Scoop the cat up so the towel or blanket encompasses the cat.

c. If you are alone, tie the ends of the towel or blanket together with cord to form a bag, or place the cat in a closed box.

d. Transport to the veterinarian.

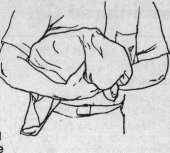

Step 2b

B. If the cat needs a stretcher

STEP 1: Use a blanket or a flat board or strong piece of cardboard. If you are using a board or piece of cardboard, proceed to STEP 2.
If you are using a blanket:

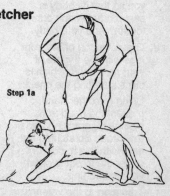

Step 1a

a. Place one hand under the cat's chest and the other hand under its rear; carefully lift or slide the cat onto the blanket.

b. Grasp each end of the blanket and lift; try to keep the blanket taut to form a stretcher.

c. Transport to the veterinarian.

CAUTION: A flat board or strong piece of cardboard must be used if a broken back is suspected.

STEP 2: If you are using a flat board or strong piece of cardboard:

a. Use a firm piece of cardboard, table leaf, TV table top, cutting board, or removable bookshelf. Make sure whatever you use will fit in your car.

b. Place two or three long strips of cloth or rope under the board, avoiding the area where the cat's neck will rest.

c. Place one hand under the cat's chest and the other under its rear; carefully lift or slide the cat onto the board.

d. Tie the cat to the board to prevent it from falling.

e. Transport to the veterinarian.

Step 2c

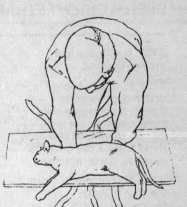

Step 2d

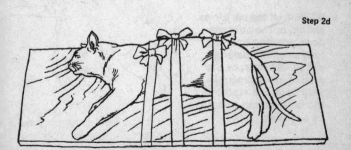

Abscess

SIGNS: SOFT, PAINFUL SWELLING; FOUL-SMELLING DISCHARGE FROM OPEN WOUND; LETHARGY.

STEP 1: Clip the hair around the area.

STEP 2: If the abscess is draining, proceed to Step 3. If not, apply hot moist compresses for 20 minute periods two or three times a day until the abscess starts draining.

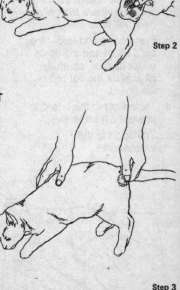

Step 2

STEP 3: Thoroughly clean the area with 3% hydrogen peroxide two or three times a day. DO NOT use any other antiseptic. Keep a scab from forming for two or three days by picking it off with your fingernail.

STEP 4: If the cat stops eating, or the abscess does not stop draining foul-smelling material within 48 hours, or the area of involvement is very large, transport to the veterinarian as soon as possible.

Step 3

Administering Oral Medicine

If the cat is hard to
handle, you will need
help restraining it.

A. Liquids

STEP 1: Restrain the cat.

a. Relieve the cat's
apprehension by talking
quietly and reassuringly;
however, be firm.

b. Grasp the skin on the
back of the neck just
below the ears and
lift the cat to a raised
surface or table that it is
unfamiliar with.

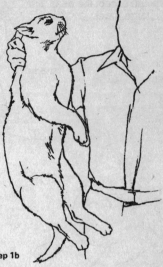

Step 1b

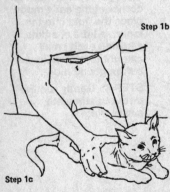

Step 1c

c. If an assistant is
necessary, have him
place both hands around
the cat's shoulders and
gently but firmly push the
cat down on the table so it
cannot use its front paws
to scratch.

continued

d. If the cat is somewhat aggressive, have an assistant wrap the entire cat, except the head, in a large towel.

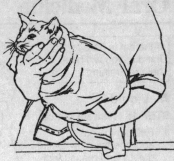

Step 1d

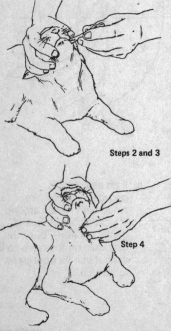

Steps 2 and 3

Step 4

STEP 2: Gently hold the cat's mouth shut and tip its head up slightly.

STEP 3: Using a plastic eye dropper or dose syringe inserted into the corner of the cat's mouth, place the fluid into the mouth a little at a time, allowing each small amount to be swallowed before giving more.

STEP 4: Gently rub the throat to stimulate swallowing.

B. Pills

> If the pill is unusually large, lubricate it with white petroleum jelly or butter.

STEP 1: Restrain the cat.

a. Relieve the cat's apprehension by talking quietly and reassuringly; however, be firm.

b. Grasp the skin on the back of the neck just below the ears and lift the cat to a raised surface or table that it is unfamiliar with.

c. If an assistant is necessary, have him place both hands around the cat's shoulders and gently but firmly push the cat down on the table so it cannot use its front paws to scratch.

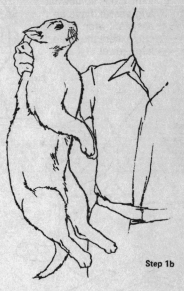

Step 1b

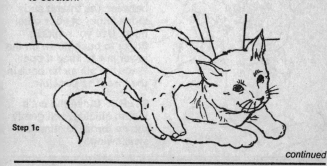

Step 1c

continued

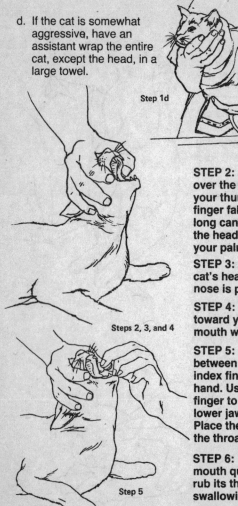

d. If the cat is somewhat aggressive, have an assistant wrap the entire cat, except the head, in a large towel.

Step 1d

Steps 2, 3, and 4

Step 5

STEP 2: Place one hand over the cat's head so that your thumb and index finger fall just behind the long canines (fang teeth), the head resting against your palm.

STEP 3: Gently tilt the cat's head back so its nose is pointing upward.

STEP 4: Push your thumb toward your finger; the mouth will open.

STEP 5: Hold the pill between the thumb and index finger of your other hand. Use your middle finger to push down on the lower jaw to keep it open. Place the pill as far back in the throat as possible.

STEP 6: Close the cat's mouth quickly, and gently rub its throat to stimulate swallowing.

Animal Bite

STEP 1: Approach the cat (see page 7); then restrain if necessary (see page 8 or 13).

STEP 2: Clip the hair around the wound.

STEP 3: Flush thoroughly by pouring 3% hydrogen peroxide into the wound. DO NOT use any other antiseptic.

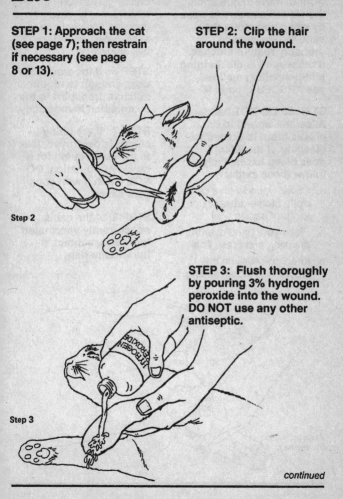

Step 2

Step 3

continued

STEP 4: Examine the wound. If the tissue under the wound appears to pass by when you move the skin, the wound will probably require stitches. If the wound is discharging a foul-smelling material, see ABSCESS, page 18.

STEP 5: DO NOT bandage. Allow the wound to drain unless there is excessive bleeding. If the wound does bleed excessively, follow these steps:

a. Cover wound with a clean cloth, sterile dressing, or sanitary napkin.

b. Place your hand over the dressing and press firmly.

c. Keep pressure on the dressing to stop bleeding.

If blood soaks through the dressing, DO NOT remove. Apply more dressing and continue to apply pressure until bleeding stops.

STEP 6: If the wound is deep enough to require stitches, transport to the veterinarian immediately.

STEP 7: If the biting animal is destroyed, take it to the veterinarian for a rabies examination. DO NOT touch it with your bare hands.

STEP 8: If the cat is not currently vaccinated for rabies, contact the veterinarian.

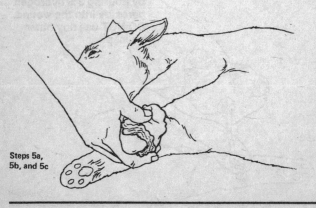

Steps 5a,
5b, and 5c

Bladder Infection

SIGNS: URINATING OUTSIDE THE LITTER PAN, STRAINING TO URINATE EVIDENCED BY GOING IN AND OUT OF LITTER PAN AND SQUATTING FOR LONG PERIODS OF TIME, BLOOD IN URINE, EXCESSIVE LICKING OF GENITAL AREA, VOMITING WITH ABOVE SIGNS.

A. If the cat is a male

STEP 1: Approach the cat (see page 7); then restrain if necessary (see page 8 or 13).

STEP 2: Check for possible obstruction of the penis, which is life-threatening.

a. Place the palm of your hand on the cat's abdomen immediately in front of the rear legs.

Step 2a

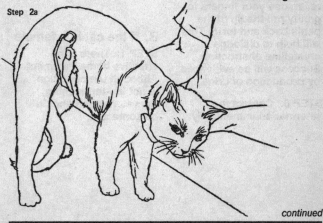

continued

b. Close your fingers toward your thumb.

c. If the cat cries out in pain or you feel a large, firm object in the abdomen, which is the distended urinary bladder, the cat is probably obstructed; proceed to Step 3. If not, proceed to Step 6.

STEP 3: Have an assistant use one hand to apply pressure over the cat's shoulders, forcing the cat firmly down, while he uses other hand to hold one or both of the back legs.

STEP 4: Lift the cat's tail to expose its hind end.

STEP 5: To provide some relief, use your fingers to gently roll the tip of the penis back and forth. This will help to dislodge crystalline obstruction. Success will be evidenced by production of urine.

STEP 6: Contact the veterinarian immediately.

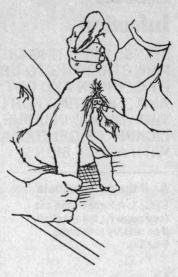

Steps 3, 4, and 5

B. If the cat is a female

STEP 1: There is no effective home treatment. Although the condition is not life-threatening, the veterinarian should be contacted.

Spurting Blood

WATCH FOR SIGNS OF SHOCK:

Pale or white gums, rapid heartbeat and breathing. If signs are present see page 118.

A. On head or torso

STEP 1: Approach the cat (see page 7); then restrain if necessary (see page 8 or 13).

STEP 2: Cover the wound with a clean folded towel, sterile gauze pad, heavy cloth, or sanitary napkin.

> If any wound is spurting blood, it means an artery has been cut. This requires immediate professional attention.

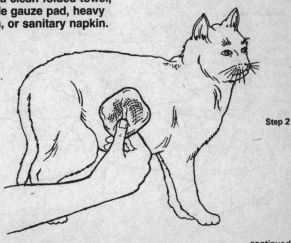

Step 2

continued

STEP 3: Wrap torn rags or other soft material around the dressing and tie or tape just tightly enough to hold in place.

STEP 4: Transport to the veterinarian immediately.

B. On legs or tail

STEP 1: Approach the cat (see page 7); then restrain if necessary (see page 8 or 13).

STEP 2: Apply a tourniquet.

a. Use a tie or piece of cloth folded to about one inch width. DO NOT use rope, wire, or string.

b. Place the material between the wound and the heart, an inch or two above, but not touching, the wound.

c. Wrap the tie or cloth twice around the appendage and cross the ends.

Steps 2b and 2c

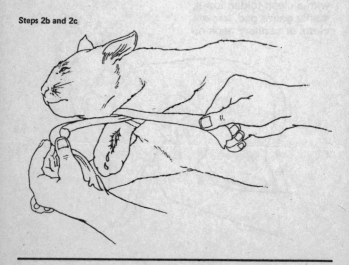

d. Tie a stick or ruler to
   the material with a
   single knot.

e. Twist the stick until
   bleeding stops,
   but no tighter.

f. Wrap a piece of cloth
   around the stick and limb
   to keep in place.

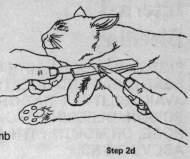

Step 2d

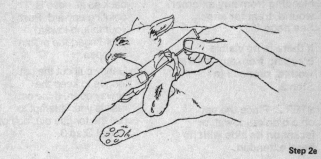

Step 2e

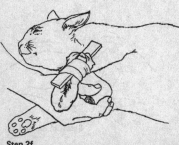

Step 2f

**STEP 3: If it will take time
to reach the veterinarian,
loosen the tourniquet
every 15 minutes
for a period of one to
two minutes and
then retighten.**

**STEP 4: Transport to the
veterinarian immediately.**

Internal Bleeding

SIGNS: PALE OR WHITE GUMS; RAPID HEARTBEAT AND BREATHING; AVAILABILITY OF RAT OR MOUSE POISON; BLEEDING FROM THE EARS, NOSE, OR MOUTH WITH ANY OF THE ABOVE SIGNS.

STEP 1: If there is bleeding from any external wound, treat for shock. See page 118.

If there is no visible bleeding from any external wound, proceed to Step 2.

STEP 2: Place the cat on a blanket, towel, or jacket on its side with its head extended.

STEP 3: Clear the airway.

a. Place one hand over the cat's head so that your thumb and index finger fall just behind the long canines (fang teeth), the head resting against your palm.

b. Gently tilt the cat's head back so its nose is pointing upward. Push your thumb toward your finger; the mouth will open.

c. Gently pull out the cat's tongue to keep the airway open. If the cat resists your attempt to pull the tongue out, do not repeat Step 3.

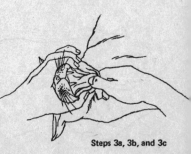

Steps 3a, 3b, and 3c

STEP 4: Elevate the cat's hindquarters slightly by placing them on a pillow or folded or rolled up towel.

STEP 5: Conserve body heat.

a. Place a hot water bottle or container (100°F/37°C) against the abdomen. Wrap the bottle in cloth to prevent burns.

b. Wrap the cat in a blanket or jacket.

STEP 6: Transport to the veterinarian immediately.

Step 4

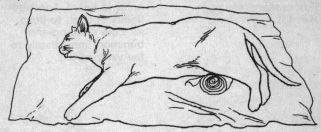

Step 5a

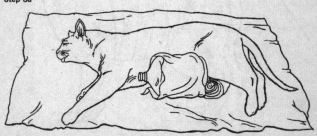

Bleeding Chest
or Abdomen

WATCH FOR
SIGNS OF SHOCK:

Pale or white gums, rapid heartbeat and breathing. If signs are present see page 118.

STEP 1: Approach the cat (see page 7); then restrain if necessary (see page 8 or 13).

STEP 2: If the wound is in the chest and a "sucking" noise is heard, bandage tightly enough to keep air from entering and transport immediately to the veterinarian.

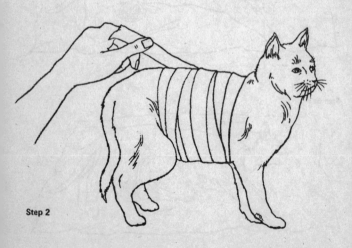

Step 2

STEP 3: If there is a
protruding object, such as
an arrow, see page 107.

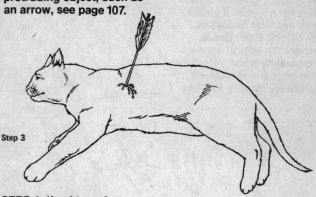

Step 3

STEP 4: If neither of
the above situations
exists, proceed to treat
the wound: clip the
hair around the
injured area.

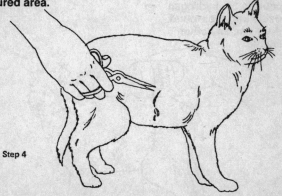

Step 4

continued

STEP 5: Examine the wound for glass or other foreign objects. If visible, remove with fingers or tweezers. If the tissue under the wound appears to pass by when you move the skin, the wound will probably require stitches.

Step 5

STEP 6: Flush thoroughly by pouring 3% hydrogen peroxide into the wound. DO NOT use any other antiseptic.

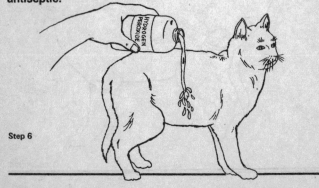

Step 6

STEP 7: Cover the wound with a clean cloth, sterile dressing, or sanitary napkin.

STEP 8: Place your hand over the dressing and press firmly.

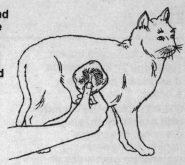

Step 7

STEP 9: Keep pressure on the dressing to stop bleeding. If blood soaks through the dressing, DO NOT remove. Apply more dressing and continue to apply pressure until bleeding stops.

STEP 10: Wrap torn sheets or other soft material around the dressing and tie or tape just tightly enough to keep it in place. Transport to the veterinarian as soon as possible.

STEP 11: If the wound is deep enough to require stitches, transport to the veterinarian immediately.

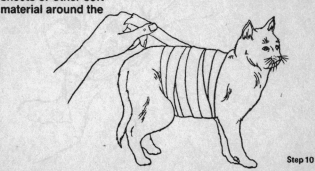

Step 10

35

Bleeding Ear

STEP 1: Approach the cat (see page 7); then restrain if necessary (see page 8 or 13).

STEP 2: Cover the wound with a clean cloth, sterile dressing, or sanitary napkin. Place dressing material on both sides of the ear flap and hold firmly to control bleeding. Cats' ears will usually stop bleeding within five minutes after pressure is applied.

STEP 3: Transport to the veterinarian immediately.

> Cut ears may bleed profusely

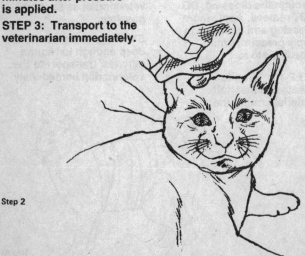

Step 2

Bleeding Leg, Paw, or Tail

WATCH FOR SIGNS OF SHOCK:

Pale or white gums, rapid heartbeat and breathing. If signs are present see page 118.

STEP 1: Approach the cat (see page 7); then restrain if necessary (see page 8 or 13).

STEP 2: Clip the hair around the injured area.

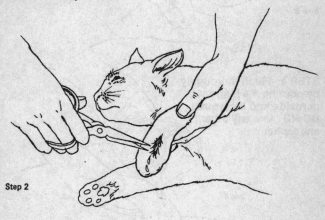

Step 2

continued

STEP 3: Examine the wound for glass or other foreign objects. If visible, remove with fingers or tweezers. If the tissue under the wound appears to pass by when you move the skin, the wound will probably require stitches.

STEP 4: Flush thoroughly by pouring 3% hydrogen peroxide into the wound. DO NOT use any other antiseptic.

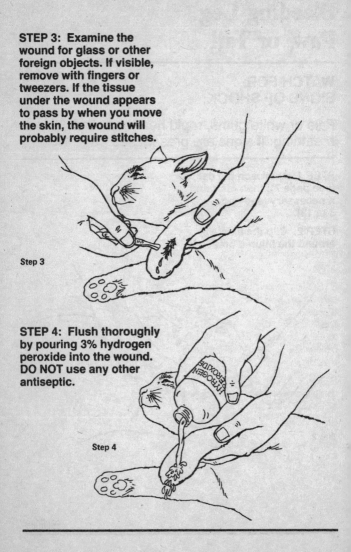

Step 3

Step 4

STEP 5: Cover the wound with a clean cloth, sterile dressing, or sanitary napkin.

STEP 6: Place your hand over the dressing and press firmly.

STEP 7: Keep pressure on the dressing to stop bleeding. If blood soaks through the dressing, DO NOT remove. Apply more dressing and continue to apply pressure until bleeding stops. If bleeding does not stop within five minutes, proceed to Step 10.

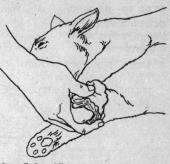

Steps 5, 6, and 7

STEP 8: Wrap torn rags or other soft material around the dressing and tie or tape just tightly enough to keep it in place. Start below the wound and wrap upward.

STEP 9: If the wound is deep enough to require stitches, keep the cat off the injured leg and transport to the veterinarian immediately.

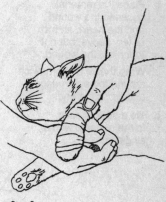

Step 8

continued

STEP 10: If bleeding does not stop within five minutes, apply a tourniquet.

Steps 10b and 10c

a. Use a tie or piece of cloth folded to about one inch width. DO NOT use rope wire, or string.

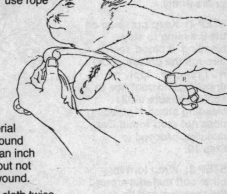

b. Place the material between the wound and the heart, an inch or two above, but not touching, the wound.

c. Wrap the tie or cloth twice around the appendage and cross the ends.

d. Tie a stick or ruler to the material with a single knot.

Step 10d

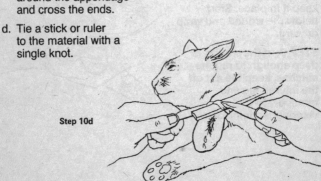

e. Twist the stick until
   bleeding stops,
   but no tighter.

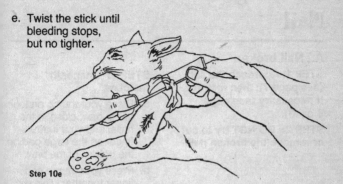

Step 10e

f. Wrap a piece of cloth
   around the stick and limb
   to keep in place.

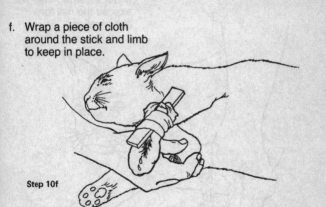

Step 10f

**STEP 11: If it will take time
to reach the veterinarian,
loosen the tourniquet
every 15 minutes for a
period of one to two
minutes and then
retighten.**

**STEP 12: Transport to the
veterinarian immediately.**

41

Bleeding Nail

A. Nail broken

STEP 1: Approach the cat (see page 7); then restrain if necessary (see page 8 or 13).

STEP 2: DO NOT try to cut or remove the broken nail.

STEP 3: Unsheath the claw.

a. Place your thumb on top of the paw, close to the nails, and your index finger on the large pad on the bottom of the paw.

b. Press your thumb and finger together. This will expose the nail for examination.

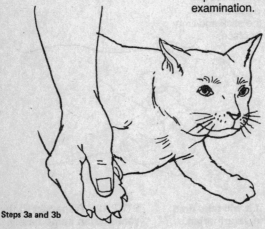

Steps 3a and 3b

STEP 4: With the nail exposed, hold a clean cloth, sterile dressing, or sanitary napkin against the nail. Bleeding will stop in a few minutes.

STEP 5: If cat seems to be in severe pain, or if bleeding does not stop in a few minutes, transport to the veterinarian as soon as possible. Continuous bleeding indicates a bleeding disorder that should be treated promptly.

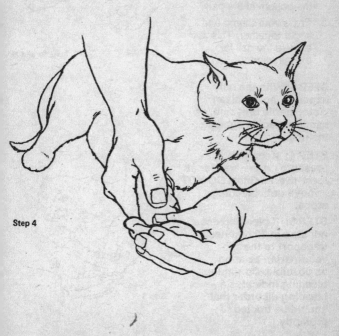

Step 4

continued

B. Nail cut too short

STEP 1: Approach the cat (see page 7); then restrain if necessary (see page 8 or 13).

STEP 2: Unsheath the claw.

a. Place your thumb on top of the paw, close to the nails, and your index finger on the large pad on the bottom of the paw.

b. Press your thumb and finger together. This will expose the nail for examination.

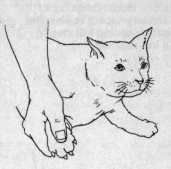

Steps 2a and 2b

STEP 3: With the nail exposed, hold a clean cloth, sterile dressing, or sanitary napkin against the nail.

STEP 4: Keep firm pressure on the area for at least five minutes. DO NOT remove until bleeding stops.

STEP 5: If bleeding does not stop in 10 minutes, transport to the veterinarian as soon as possible. Continuous bleeding indicates a bleeding disorder that should be treated promptly.

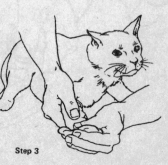

Step 3

Bleeding Nose

STEP 1: Approach the cat (see page 7); then restrain if necessary (see page 8 or 13).

STEP 2: Apply an ice pack to the top of the cat's nose between its eyes and nostrils.

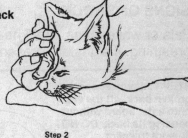

Step 2

STEP 3: Cover the bleeding nostril with a clean cloth, sterile dressing, or sanitary napkin.

STEP 4: Hold firmly until bleeding stops.

STEP 5: If the nostril was not cut, a bloody nose in a cat could indicate a serious disorder. Transport to the veterinarian as soon as possible.

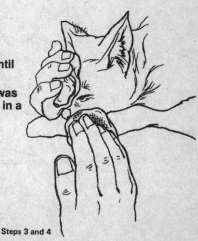

Steps 3 and 4

Broken Back

SIGNS: EXTREME PAIN IN SPINE AREA, UNUSUAL ARCH TO SPINE, PARALYSIS.

**WATCH FOR
SIGNS OF SHOCK:**

Pale or white gums, rapid heartbeat and breathing. If signs are present see page 118.

STEP 1: If you suspect a broken back, lift the cat onto a flat board without bending its back. DO NOT attempt to splint.

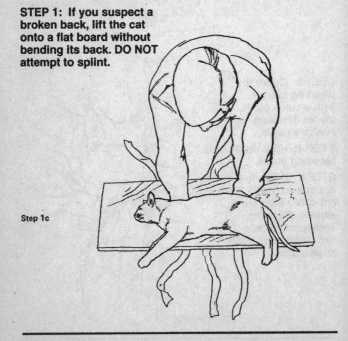

Step 1c

a. Use a firm piece of cardboard, table leaf, TV table top, cutting board, or removable bookshelf. Make sure whatever you use will fit in your car.

b. Place two or three long strips of cloth or rope under the board, avoiding the area where the cat's neck will rest.

c. Place one hand under the cat's chest and the other under its rear; carefully lift or slide the cat onto the board.

d. Tie the cat to the board to prevent it from falling.

STEP 2: Transport to the veterinarian immediately.

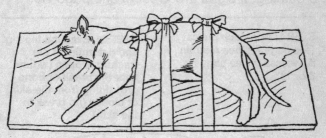

Step 1d

47

Broken Leg

SIGNS: LEG IS MISSHAPEN, HANGS LIMPLY, CANNOT SUPPORT BODY WEIGHT; SUDDEN ONSET OF PAIN IN AREA; SWELLING.

WATCH FOR SIGNS OF SHOCK:

Pale or white gums, rapid heartbeat and breathing. If signs are present see page 118.

STEP 1: Approach the cat (see page 7); then restrain if necessary (see page 8 or 13).

STEP 2: Examine the leg and determine if the fracture is open (wound near the break or bone protruding from the skin) or closed (no break in the skin).

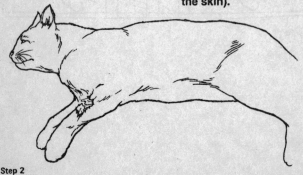

Step 2
Open Fracture

STEP 3: If the fracture is closed, proceed to Step 4.

If the fracture is open:

a. Flush thoroughly by
   pouring 3% hydrogen
   peroxide into the wound.
   DO NOT use any other
   antiseptic.

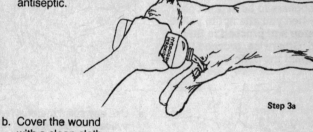

Step 3a

b. Cover the wound
   with a clean cloth,
   sterile dressing, or
   sanitary napkin.

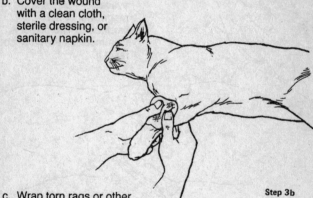

Step 3b

c. Wrap torn rags or other
   soft material around
   the dressing and tie or
   tape just tightly enough to
   keep it in place.

continued

d. DO NOT attempt to splint the fracture. Hold a folded towel under the unsplinted limb and transport to the veterinarian immediately.

STEP 4: If the limb with the closed fracture is grossly misshapen or the cat appears to be in great pain when you attempt to splint, stop and proceed to Step 5. Otherwise, proceed to splint the bone.

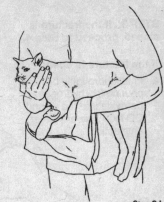

Step 3d

a. Use any splint material available—sticks, a magazine, or stiff cardboard. The object is to immobilize the limb, not reset it.

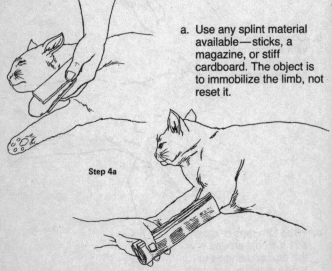

Step 4a

b. Tie splints to the fractured leg with torn strips of cloth or gauze.

c. Tape or tie firmly, but not so tightly that circulation may be impaired.

d. Transport to the veterinarian immediately.

Steps 4b and 4c

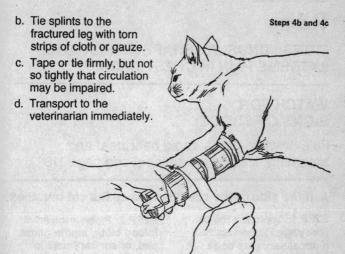

Step 5

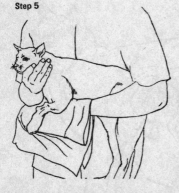

STEP 5: If the limb is grossly misshapen, or if the cat appears to be in great pain when you attempt to splint, hold a folded towel under the unsplinted limb and transport to the veterinarian immediately.

Broken Ribs

SIGNS: UNUSUAL SHAPE OF RIBCAGE, EXTREME PAIN IN CHEST AREA.

**WATCH FOR
SIGNS OF SHOCK:**

Pale or white gums, rapid heartbeat and breathing. If signs are present see page 118.

A. If the side of the chest bulges as the cat breathes

STEP 1: Approach the cat (see page 7); then restrain if necessary (see page 8 or 13).

STEP 2: Place a thick folded cloth, sterile gauze pad, or sanitary napkin over the bulge.

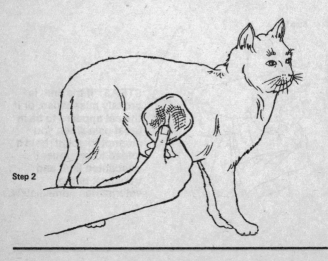

Step 2

STEP 3: Bandage with torn cloth or gauze, just tightly enough to keep pressure on the bulge.

A bulging chest usually means there is deep muscle damage to the chest wall. This requires immediate professional attention.

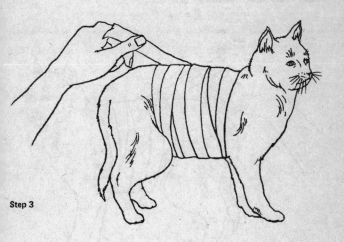

Step 3

STEP 4: Transport to the veterinarian immediately.

continued

B. If broken ribs are obvious or suspected

STEP 1: Approach the cat (see page 7); then restrain if necessary (see page 8 or 13).

STEP 3: Transport to the veterinarian immediately.

STEP 2: Wrap torn sheets or gauze around the entire chest area to immobilize.

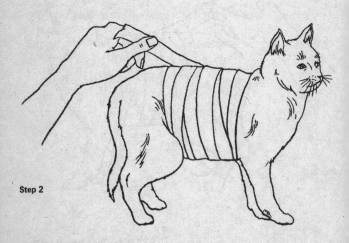

Step 2

First or Second Degree Burns

SIGNS: FIRST DEGREE—FUR INTACT OR SINGED, PAINFUL LESION, SKIN RED WITH POSSIBLE BLISTERS.

SECOND DEGREE—SINGED FUR, PAINFUL LESION WHICH TURNS DRY AND TAN, SWELLING.

STEP 1: Approach the cat (see page 7); then restrain if necessary (see page 8 or 13).

STEP 2: Apply cold water or ice packs to the burned area; leave in contact with the skin for 15 minutes. DO NOT apply ointment or butter.

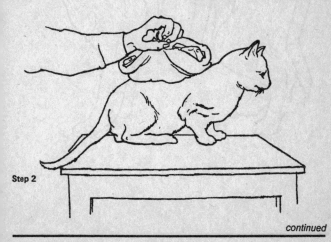

Step 2

continued

STEP 3: If burns cover a large part of the body or are located where the cat can lick them, cover with a sterile dressing. DO NOT use cotton.

STEP 4: Wrap torn rags or other soft material around the dressing and tie or tape just tightly enough to keep it in place.

STEP 5: Transport to the veterinarian as soon as possible.

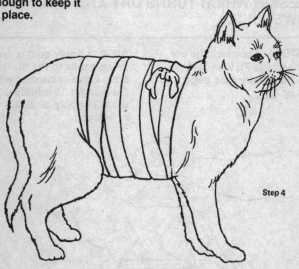

Step 4

Third
Degree Burns

SIGNS: PROBABLE SHOCK IF EXTENSIVE BODY AREA IS INVOLVED, DESTRUCTION OF ENTIRE SKIN AREA, BLACK OR PURE WHITE LESION, FUR PULLS OUT EASILY.

**WATCH FOR
SIGNS OF SHOCK:**

Pale or white gums, rapid heartbeat and breathing. If signs are present see page 118.

STEP 1: Approach the cat (see page 7); then restrain if necessary (see page 8 or 13).

STEP 2: Apply a sterile dressing over the burned area. DO NOT use cotton.

STEP 3: Wrap torn rags or other soft material around the dressing and tie or tape just tightly enough to keep it in place.

STEP 4: Transport to the veterinarian immediately.

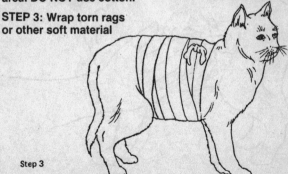

Step 3

Chemical Burns

SIGNS: CHEMICAL ODOR SUCH AS TURPENTINE, GASOLINE, OR INSECTICIDE; REDDENED SKIN; PAIN.

STEP 1: Approach the cat (see page 7); then restrain if necessary (see page 8 or 13).

STEP 2: Wash the area thoroughly with mild soap or shampoo and water. Lather well and rinse thoroughly. Repeat as many times as necessary to remove the chemical. DO NOT use solvents of any kind.

STEP 3: Apply a soothing antibiotic ointment to the affected area.

STEP 4: Call the veterinarian for further instructions.

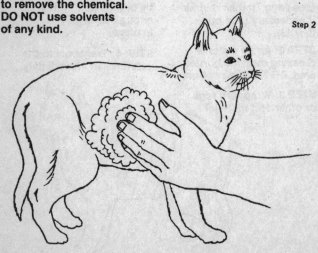

Step 2

Choking

SIGNS: PAWING AT MOUTH, PALE OR BLUE TONGUE, OBVIOUS DISTRESS, UNCONSCIOUSNESS.

STEP 1: Approach the cat (see page 7); then restrain if necessary (see page 8 or 13).

STEP 2: Clear the airway.

a. Place one hand over the cat's head so that your thumb and index finger fall just behind the long canines (fang teeth), the head resting against your palm. If the cat is struggling too much, proceed to Step 2e.

b. Gently tilt the cat's head back so its nose is pointing upward. Push your thumb toward your finger; the mouth will open.

c. Gently pull the tongue out. If you can see the object, try to remove it with your fingers or needle-nose pliers (unless object is a needle).

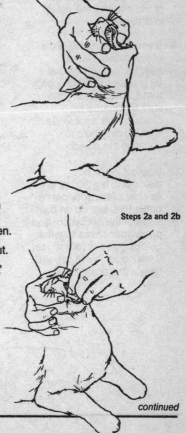

Steps 2a and 2b

Step 2c

continued

d. If object is a needle and it is embedded deeply into the roof of the mouth, stop. Transport immediately to the veterinarian. Keep the tongue gently pulled out of the mouth if the cat is in distress.

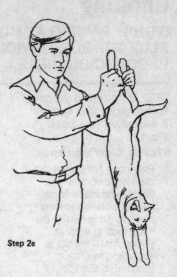

e. If you cannot remove the object (other than a needle), pick up the cat by grasping its back legs; turn it upside down and shake vigorously. Slapping the back while shaking may help to dislodge the object.

Step 2e

f. If object is still not dislodged, lay the cat on its side, place your palms behind the last rib on both sides of the abdomen, and press your palms together quickly three or four times. If the object is still caught, repeat this procedure.

STEP 3: If you cannot dislodge the object, transport to the veterinarian immediately.

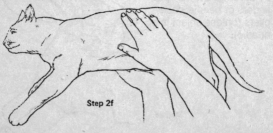

Step 2f

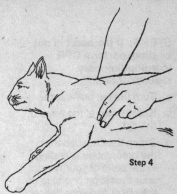

STEP 4: If you dislodge the object but the cat is not breathing, feel for heartbeat by placing fingers about one inch behind the cat's elbow and in the center of its chest.

Step 4

STEP 5: If the heart is not beating, proceed to Step 6. If it is beating, perform artificial respiration.

a. Turn the cat on its side.

b. Hold the cat's mouth and lips closed and blow firmly into its nostrils. Blow for three seconds, take a deep breath, and repeat until you feel resistance or see the chest rise.

c. After one minute, stop. Watch the chest for movement to indicate the cat is breathing on its own.

d. If the cat is still not breathing, continue artificial respiration.

e. Transport to the veterinarian immediately and continue artificial respiration on the way to the veterinarian or until the cat is breathing without assistance.

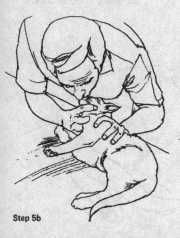

Step 5b

continued

STEP 6: If the heart is not beating, perform CPR (cardiopulmonary resuscitation).

a. Turn the cat on its side.

b. Kneel down at the head of the cat.

c. Grasp the chest so that the breastbone is resting in the palm of your hand, your thumb on one side of the chest and your fingers on the other. Your thumb and fingers should fall in the middle of the chest.

d. Compress the chest by firmly squeezing your thumb and fingers together for a count of "two" and release for a count of "one." Repeat about 30 times in 30 seconds.

e. Alternately (after 30 seconds), hold the cat's mouth and lips closed and blow firmly into its nostrils. Blow for three seconds, take a deep breath, and repeat until you feel resistance or see the chest rise. Repeat this 20 times in 60 seconds.

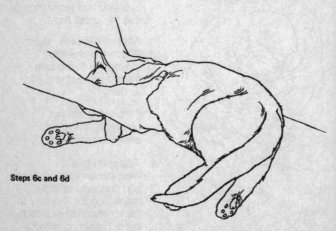

Steps 6c and 6d

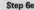

Step 6e

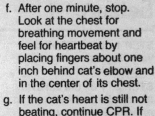

f. After one minute, stop. Look at the chest for breathing movement and feel for heartbeat by placing fingers about one inch behind cat's elbow and in the center of its chest.

g. If the cat's heart is still not beating, continue CPR. If the heart starts beating, but the cat is still not breathing, return to Step 5b to continue artificial respiration.

STEP 7: Transport to the veterinarian immediately. CPR or artificial respiration should be continued on the way or until the cat is breathing and its heart is beating without assistance.

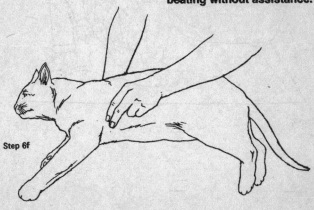

Step 6f

Convulsion/ Seizure

STEP 1: DO NOT place your fingers or any object in the cat's mouth.

STEP 2: Pull the cat away from walls and furniture to prevent self-injury.

Be patient; do not panic. Convulsions are rarely fatal and most last only a few minutes.

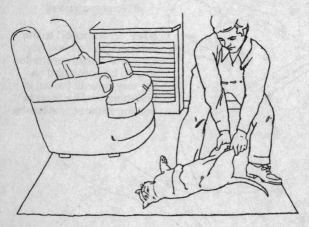

Step 2

STEP 3: Wrap the cat in a blanket to help protect it from injury.

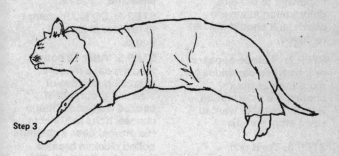

Step 3

STEP 4: When the seizure has stopped, contact the veterinarian for further instructions.

STEP 5: If the seizure does not stop within 10 minutes, or if the cat comes out of the seizure and goes into another one within an hour, transport to the veterinarian immediately.

STEP 6: Expect the cat to be dazed and very frightened for 10 to 15 minutes after the seizure.

Diarrhea

STEP 1: Remove all food immediately. Water is important to prevent dehydration in severe diarrhea. It should not be removed.

STEP 2: If blood appears or if diarrhea continues for more than 24 hours, contact the veterinarian. He will probably want to see a stool sample.

STEP 3: Treat with Kaopectate® every four to six hours at the rate of ½ teaspoon per five to seven pounds of the cat's weight. See Administering Oral Medicine, page 19.

STEP 4: DO NOT attempt to feed for at least 12 hours.

STEP 5: After 12 hours, feed the cat a mixture of small quantities of steamed ground beef, cooked rice, and cottage cheese. If the cat rejects the ground beef, substitute boiled chicken breasts, skinned and boned. This diet should be continued until stools are formed.

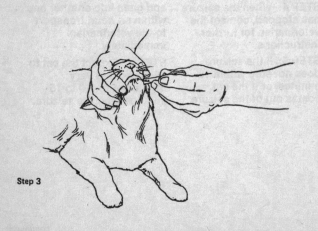

Step 3

Drowning

STEP 1: Rescue the cat.

a. Holding a rope attached to a life preserver, throw the preserver toward the cat. OR

b. Try to hook the cat's collar with a pole. OR

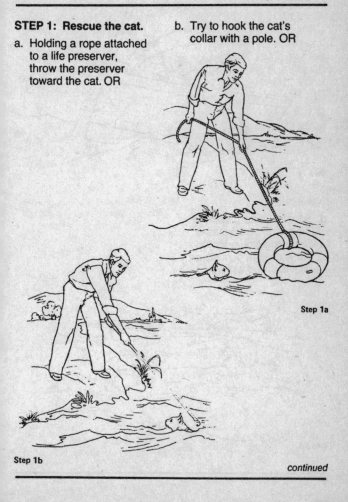

Step 1a

Step 1b

continued

c. Row out to the cat in a boat. OR

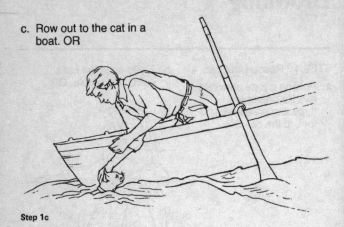

Step 1c

d. As a last resort, swim to the cat. Protect yourself. Bring something for the cat to cling to or climb on as it is pulled ashore.

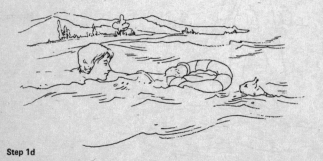

Step 1d

STEP 2: Drain the lungs. Grasp the rear legs and hold the animal upside down for 15–20 seconds. Give three or four downward shakes to help drain fluid from the lungs.

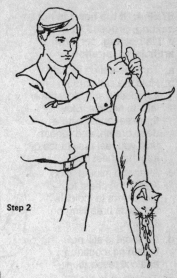

Step 2

STEP 3: If the cat is not breathing, feel for heartbeat by placing fingers about one inch behind the cat's elbow and in the center of its chest.

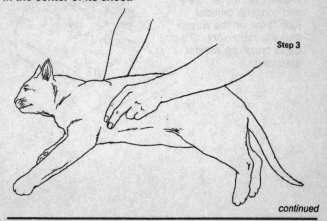

Step 3

continued

STEP 4: If the heart is not beating, proceed to Step 5. If it is beating, perform artificial respiration.

a. Turn the cat on its side.

b. Hold the cat's mouth and lips closed and blow firmly into its nostrils. Blow for three seconds, take a deep breath, and repeat until you feel resistance or see the chest rise.

c. After one minute, stop. Watch the chest for movement to indicate the cat is breathing on its own.

d. If the cat is still not breathing, continue artificial respiration.

e. Transport to the veterinarian immediately and continue artificial respiration on the way to the veterinarian or until the cat is breathing without assistance.

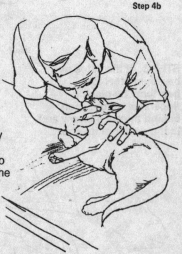

Step 4b

STEP 5: If the heart is not beating, perform CPR (cardiopulmonary resuscitation).

a. Turn the cat on its side.

b. Kneel down at the head of the cat.

c. Grasp the chest so that the breastbone is resting in the palm of your hand, your thumb on one side of the chest and your fingers on the other. Your thumb and fingers should fall in the middle of the chest.

d. Compress the chest by firmly squeezing your thumb and fingers together for a count of "two" and release for a count of "one." Repeat about 30 times in 30 seconds.

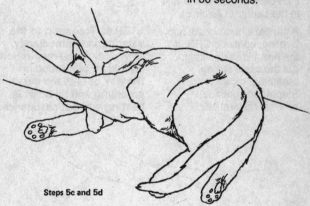

Steps 5c and 5d

continued

e. Alternately (after 30 seconds), hold the cat's mouth and lips closed and blow firmly into its nostrils. Blow for three seconds, take a deep breath, and repeat until you feel resistance or see the chest rise. Repeat this 20 times in 60 seconds.

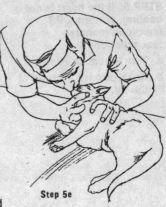

Step 5e

f. After one minute, stop. Look at the chest for breathing movement and feel for heartbeat by placing fingers about one inch behind cat's elbow and in the center of its chest.

g. If the cat's heart is still not beating, continue CPR. If the heart starts beating, but the cat is still not breathing, return to Step 4b to continue artificial respiration.

STEP 6: Transport to the veterinarian immediately. CPR or artificial respiration should be continued on the way or until the cat is breathing and its heart is beating without assistance.

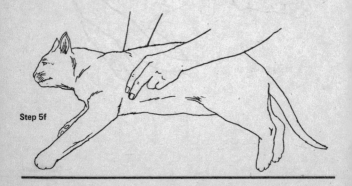

Step 5f

Electrical Shock

WATCH FOR SIGNS OF SHOCK:

Pale or white gums, rapid heartbeat and breathing. If signs are present see page 118.

STEP 1: If the cat still has the electric cord in its mouth, DO NOT touch. First remove the plug from its outlet.

Step 1

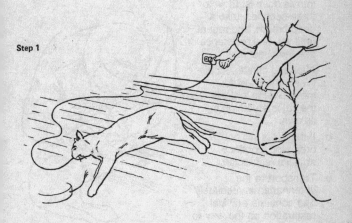

continued

STEP 2: If the cat is breathing, proceed to Step 6. If the cat is not breathing, feel for heartbeat by placing fingers about one inch behind the cat's elbow and in the center of its chest.

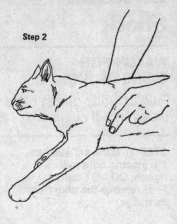

Step 2

STEP 3: If the heart is not beating, proceed to Step 4. If it is beating, perform artificial respiration.

a. Turn the cat on its side.

b. Hold the cat's mouth and lips closed and blow firmly into its nostrils. Blow for three seconds, take a deep breath, and repeat until you feel resistance or see the chest rise.

c. After one minute, stop. Watch the chest for movement to indicate the cat is breathing on its own.

d. If the cat is still not breathing, continue artificial respiration.

e. Transport to the veterinarian immediately and continue artificial respiration on the way to the veterinarian or until the cat is breathing without assistance.

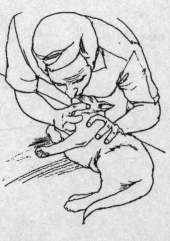

Step 3b

STEP 4: If the heart is not beating, perform CPR (cardiopulmonary resuscitation).

a. Turn the cat on its side.

b. Kneel down at the head of the cat.

c. Grasp the chest so that the breastbone is resting in the palm of your hand, your thumb on one side of the chest and your fingers on the other. Your thumb and fingers should fall about in the middle of the chest.

d. Compress the chest by firmly squeezing your thumb and fingers together for a count of "two" and release for a count of "one." Repeat about 30 times in 30 seconds.

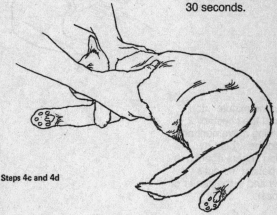

Steps 4c and 4d

continued

e. Alternately (after 30 seconds), hold the cat's mouth and lips closed and blow firmly into its nostrils. Blow for three seconds, take a deep breath, and repeat until you feel resistance or see the chest rise. Try to repeat this 20 times in 60 seconds.

Step 4e

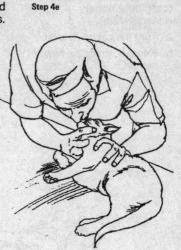

f. After one minute, stop. Look at the chest for breathing movement and feel for heartbeat by placing fingers about one inch behind the cat's elbow and in the center of its chest.

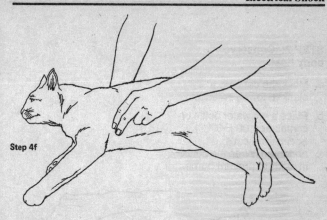

Step 4f

g. If the cat's heart is still not beating, continue CPR. If the heart starts beating, but the cat is still not breathing, return to Step 3b to continue artificial respiration.

STEP 5: Transport to the veterinarian immediately. CPR or artificial respiration should be continued on the way to the veterinarian or until the cat is breathing and its heart is beating without assistance.

STEP 6: If the cat's mouth or lips are burned (bright red), swab them gently with 3% hydrogen peroxide. DO NOT use any other antiseptic.

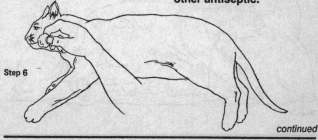

Step 6

continued

STEP 7: Conserve body heat.

a. Move the cat onto a blanket, towel, or jacket.

b. Place a hot water bottle or container (100°F/37°C) against the cat's abdomen. Wrap the bottle in cloth to prevent burns.

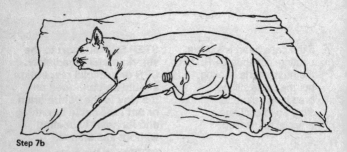

Step 7b

c. Wrap the cat in a blanket or jacket.

STEP 8: Transport to the veterinarian immediately.

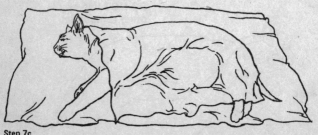

Step 7c

Object in Eye

STEP 1: DO NOT try to remove the object.

STEP 2: Approach the cat (see page 7); then restrain if necessary (see page 8 or 13).

STEP 3: Prevent self-injury to the eye.

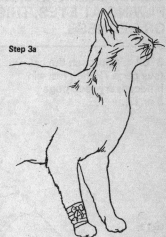

Step 3a

a. Dewclaw should be bandaged on the front paw on the same side as the affected eye.

b. If the cat is scratching at the eye continuously, cut a large piece of cardboard into an Elizabethan-type collar.

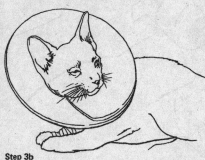

Step 3b

STEP 4: Transport to the veterinarian immediately.

Scratched or Irritated Eye

SIGNS: SQUINTING, RUBBING OR PAWING AT EYES; THICK DISCHARGE; OR REDNESS.

STEP 1: Approach the cat (see page 7); then restrain if necessary (see page 8 or 13).

STEP 2: Flush thoroughly (three or four times) by pouring dilute boric acid solution or plain water into the eye.

Step 2

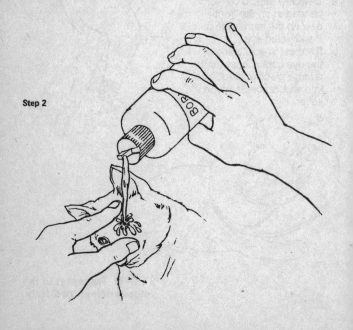

STEP 3: Prevent self-injury to the eye.

a. Dewclaw should be bandaged on the front paw on the same side as the affected eye.

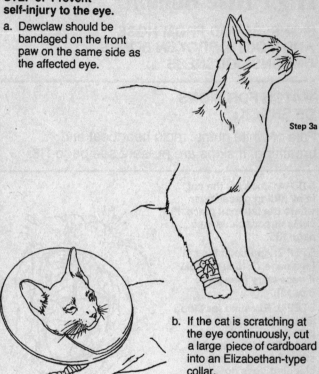

Step 3a

Step 3b

b. If the cat is scratching at the eye continuously, cut a large piece of cardboard into an Elizabethan-type collar.

STEP 4: Transport to the veterinarian immediately.

Fall from High-Rise Building

SIGNS: BLOOD FROM NOSE AND MOUTH, BROKEN BONES, UNCONSCIOUSNESS.

WATCH FOR SIGNS OF SHOCK:

Pale or white gums, rapid heartbeat and breathing. If signs are present see page 118.

STEP 1: Look for the cat in all hiding places near where the fall took place. If cat is unconscious, see page 135.

STEP 2: Approach the cat (see page 7); then restrain if necessary (see page 8 or 13).

STEP 3: Examine for blood around the nose. If present, carefully wipe away. Bleeding should stop in a few minutes. If bleeding does not stop, see BLEEDING NOSE, page 45.

STEP 4: Examine for blood, broken teeth, and/or split upper palate in mouth. To open the mouth:

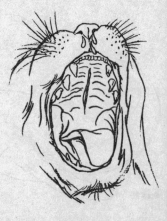

Step 4   Split Upper Palate

a. Place one hand over the cat's head so that your thumb and index finger fall just behind the long canines (fang teeth), the head resting against your palm.

b. Gently tilt the cat's head back so its nose is pointing upward. Push your thumb toward your finger; the mouth will open.

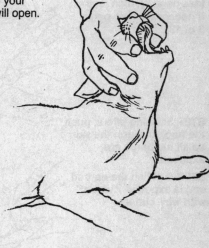

Steps 4a and 4b

STEP 5: Carefully wipe blood away from mouth; bleeding should stop in a few minutes.

STEP 6: Examine for broken bones. See pages 46, 48, and 52.

STEP 7: Transport to the veterinarian immediately.

Fish Hook Embedded in Cat

STEP 1: If the hook is in the tongue or roof of the mouth, or near the eye, DO NOT attempt to remove it; transport to the veterinarian immediately.

STEP 2: Approach the cat (see page 7); then restrain if necessary (see page 8 or 13).

STEP 3: Using pliers, push the hook through the skin so all the barbs are exposed.

STEP 4: When the barbed end is exposed, cut it off with wire cutters.

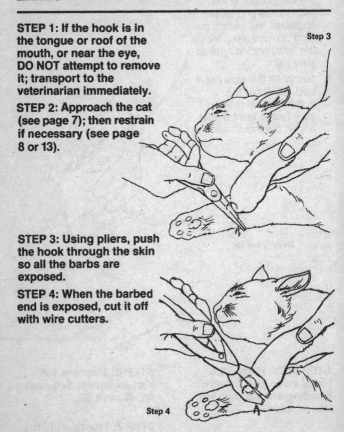

Step 3

Step 4

A

STEP 5: After the barbs have been removed, pull the hook back through the way it entered.

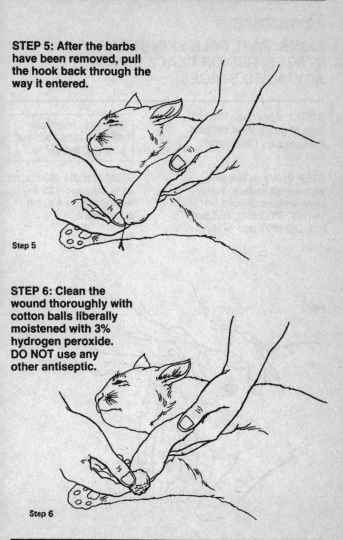

Step 5

STEP 6: Clean the wound thoroughly with cotton balls liberally moistened with 3% hydrogen peroxide. DO NOT use any other antiseptic.

Step 6

Frostbite

SIGNS: PAIN, PALE SKIN IN EARLY STAGES, RED OR BLACK SKIN IN ADVANCED STAGES.

STEP 1: Approach the cat (see page 7); then restrain if necessary (see page 8 or 13).

The most commonly affected areas are the ears and the tail tip.

STEP 2: Warm the area with moist towels. Water temperature should be warm (75°F/24°C), but not hot. DO NOT use ointment.

STEP 3: If the skin turns dark, transport to the veterinarian as soon as possible.

Step 2

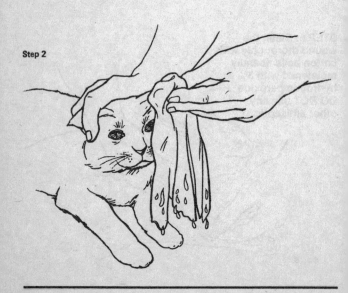

Hairball

SIGNS: CAT VOMITS UP LONG CIGAR-SHAPED MATERIAL FULL OF HAIR; VOMITS FOOD IMMEDIATELY AFTER EATING AND ATTEMPTS TO EAT AGAIN; PASSES HAIR IN STOOL; RARELY, LACK OF APPETITE AND WEIGHT LOSS.

STEP 1: Remove all food and water immediately.

STEP 2: If vomited material is bloody or has a foul odor, contact the veterinarian immediately. If not, proceed to Step 3.

STEP 3: Treat by placing one or two teaspoons of white petroleum jelly on the cat's mouth and paws so it can lick it off. DO NOT give mineral oil.

STEP 4: Repeat the petroleum jelly treatment once a day while the cat is having difficulty. If problem lasts more than two or three days, contact the veterinarian as soon as possible.

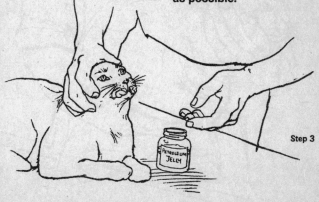

Step 3

Heart Muscle Disease

SIGNS: DIFFICULT BREATHING, LACK OF COORDINATION OR PARALYSIS OF REAR LIMBS, EXCESSIVE CRYING WITH ABOVE SIGNS.

STEP 1: Carefully wrap the cat in a blanket or towel so it feels secure.

STEP 2: There is no effective home treatment. The situation is life-threatening, and the cat should be taken to the veterinarian immediately.

Step 1

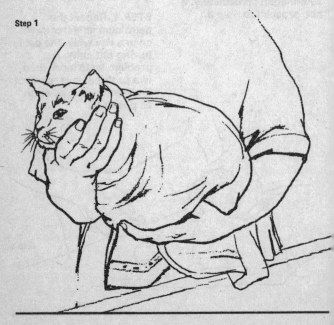

Heatstroke

SIGNS: EXCESSIVE DROOLING, LACK OF COORDINATION, RAPID BREATHING, TOP OF THE HEAD HOT TO THE TOUCH.

STEP 1: Remove the cat from the hot environment.

STEP 2: Immerse the cat in a cold water bath or continuously run a garden hose on its body; continue either treatment for at least 30 minutes.

Prompt treatment is urgent. Heatstroke can lead to brain damage and death.

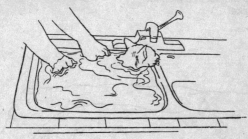

Step 2

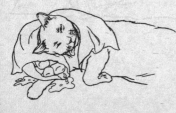

Step 3

STEP 3: Apply ice packs around the head; keep them there while transporting to the veterinarian.

STEP 4: Transport to the veterinarian immediately after the above treatment.

Hypothermia

SIGNS: DEPRESSION, SUBNORMAL BODY TEMPERATURE, COMA.

STEP 1: Warm the cat.

a. Move the cat onto a blanket, towel, or jacket.

b. Place a hot water bottle or container (100°F/37°C) against the cat's abdomen. Wrap the bottle in cloth to prevent burns. Wrap the cat in a blanket or jacket.

STEP 2: Transport to the veterinarian immediately. Continue to warm the cat during transportation.

Step 1b

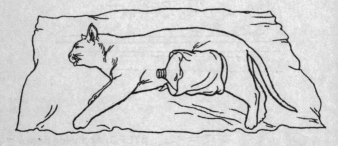

Insect Sting or Spider Bite

SIGNS: SWELLING, PAIN IN MUSCLES AND AFFECTED AREA, VOMITING, WEAKNESS, FEVER, SHOCK.

WATCH FOR SIGNS OF SHOCK:

Pale or white gums, rapid heartbeat and breathing. If signs are present see page 118.

STEP 1: Approach the cat (see page 7); then restrain if necessary (see page 8 or 13).

STEP 2: DO NOT pinch the area. If stung by a bee, scrape the stinger off immediately with a credit card or dull knife. Others do not leave the stinger in the skin.

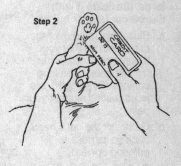

Step 2

Bee, wasp, yellow jacket, and hornet stings may produce an allergic reaction. Scorpion stings and tarantula, black widow, and brown recluse spider bites will almost certainly produce an allergic reaction.

continued

STEP 3: Apply ice cube or pack to the affected area.

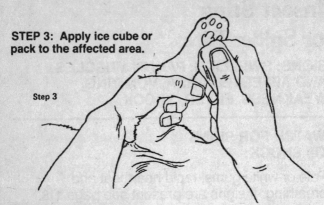

Step 3

STEP 4: Administer any single-strength cold tablet or hay fever product that contains an antihistamine; ½ tablet per seven to ten pounds of the cat's weight. If the pill is unusually large, lubricate it with petroleum jelly or butter.

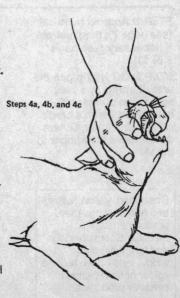

Steps 4a, 4b, and 4c

a. Place one hand over the cat's head so that your thumb and index finger fall just behind the long canines (fang teeth), the head resting against your palm.

b. Gently tilt the cat's head back so its nose is pointing upward.

c. Push your thumb toward your finger; the mouth will open.

d. Hold the pill between the thumb and index finger of your other hand. Use your middle finger to push down on the lower jaw to keep it open. Place the pill as far back in the throat as possible.

Step 4d

e. Close the cat's mouth quickly, and gently rub its throat to stimulate swallowing.

Step 4e

STEP 5: Transport to the veterinarian immediately.

Corrosive or Petroleum-Base Poisoning

SIGNS: BURNS ON MOUTH IF CORROSIVE, CHARACTERISTIC ODOR IF PETROLEUM PRODUCT, SEVERE ABDOMINAL PAIN, VOMITING, DIARRHEA, BLOODY URINE, CONVULSIONS, COMA.

WATCH FOR SIGNS OF SHOCK:

Pale or white gums, rapid heartbeat and breathing. If signs are present see page 118.

Corrosives include battery acid, corn and callous remover, dishwasher detergent, drain cleaner, grease remover, lye, and oven cleaner. Petroleum products include paint solvent, floor wax, and dry cleaning solution. If in doubt as to type of poison, call your veterinarian or local Poison Control Center.

STEP 1: If the cat is comatose or convulsing, wrap it in a blanket and take the cat and container of suspected poison to the veterinarian immediately.

STEP 2: Approach the cat (see page 7); then restrain if necessary (see page 8 or 13).

STEP 3: Flush the cat's mouth and muzzle thoroughly with large amounts of water. Hold its head at a slight downward angle so it does not choke.

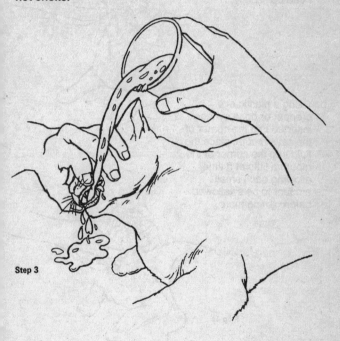

Step 3

continued

STEP 4: DO NOT induce vomiting. Give one teaspoon of olive oil or egg whites.

Steps 4a and 4b

a. Gently hold the cat's mouth shut and tip its head up slightly.

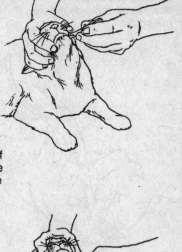

b. Using a plastic eye — dropper or dose syringe inserted into the corner of the cat's mouth, place the fluid into the corner of the mouth a little at a time, allowing each small amount to be swallowed before giving more.

Step 4c

c. Gently rub the throat to stimulate swallowing.

STEP 5: Take the cat and container of suspected poison to the veterinarian immediately.

Noncorrosive Poisoning

SIGNS: EXCESSIVE DROOLING, VOMITING, ABDOMINAL PAIN, LACK OF COORDINATION, CONVULSIONS, COMA.

WATCH FOR SIGNS OF SHOCK:

Pale or white gums, rapid heartbeat and breathing. If signs are present see page 118.

STEP 1: If the cat is comatose or convulsing, wrap it in a blanket and take the cat and container of suspected poison to the veterinarian immediately.

STEP 2: Approach the cat (see page 7); then restrain if necessary (see page 8 or 13).

STEP 3: If the cat has not already vomited, induce vomiting immediately by giving one teaspoon of 3% hydrogen peroxide every 10 minutes until the cat vomits.

a. Gently hold the cat's mouth shut and tip its head up slightly.

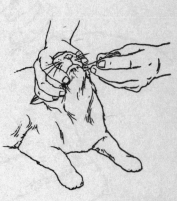

Steps 3a and 3b

continued

b. Using a plastic eye–dropper or dose syringe inserted into the corner of the cat's mouth, place the fluid into the corner of the mouth a little at a time, allowing each small amount to be swallowed before giving more.

c. Gently rub the throat to stimulate swallowing.

STEP 4: Save the vomit for the veterinarian.

STEP 5: Take the cat, vomit, and container of suspected poison to the veterinarian immediately.

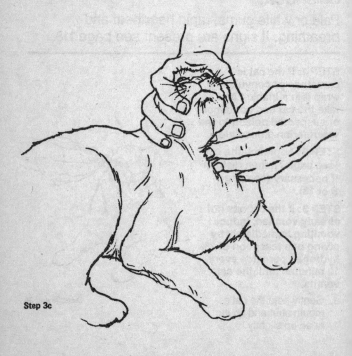

Step 3c

Poisonous Plants

SIGNS: DROOLING, VOMITING, DIARRHEA, ABDOMINAL PAIN, LACK OF COORDINATION, DIFFICULTY IN BREATHING, CONVULSIONS.

STEP 1: Approach the cat (see page 7); then restrain if necessary (see page 8 or 13).

STEP 2: If the cat has not already vomited, induce vomiting immediately by giving one teaspoon of 3% hydrogen peroxide every 10 minutes until the cat vomits.

It is safe to assume that all common house plants are toxic to some degree.

a. Gently hold the cat's mouth shut and tip its head up slightly.

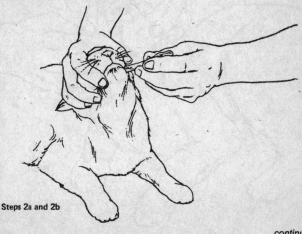

Steps 2a and 2b

continued

b. Using a plastic eye — dropper or dose syringe inserted into the corner of the cat's mouth, place the fluid into the corner of the mouth a little at a time, allowing each small amount to be swallowed before giving more.

c. Gently rub the throat to stimulate swallowing.

STEP 3: If convulsions or difficulty in breathing develops, take the cat and a leaf of the suspected plant to the veterinarian immediately.

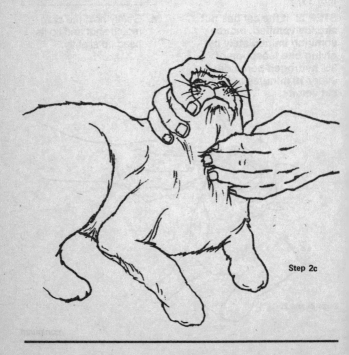

Step 2c

Smoke or Carbon Monoxide Inhalation

SIGNS: DEPRESSION, LACK OF COORDINATION, HEAVY PANTING, DEEP RED GUMS, POSSIBLE CONVULSIONS.

WATCH FOR SIGNS OF SHOCK:

Pale or white gums, rapid heartbeat and breathing. If signs are present see page 118.

A. If conscious

STEP 1: Remove the cat to fresh air immediately.

STEP 2: Flush the cat's eyes thoroughly by pouring dilute boric acid solution or plain water directly into them.

STEP 3: Transport to the veterinarian immediately.

Step 2

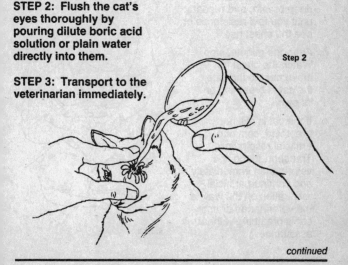

continued

B. If unconscious

STEP 1: Remove the cat to fresh air immediately.

STEP 2: If the cat is not breathing, feel for heartbeat by placing fingers about one inch behind the cat's elbow and in the center of its chest.

STEP 3: If the heart is not beating, proceed to Step 4. If it is beating, perform artificial respiration.

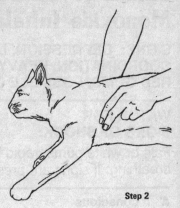

Step 2

a. Turn the cat on its side.

b. Hold the cat's mouth and lips closed and blow firmly into its nostrils. Blow for three seconds, take a deep breath, and repeat until you feel resistance or see the chest rise.

c. After one minute, stop. Watch the chest for movement to indicate the cat is breathing on its own.

d. If the cat is still not breathing, continue artificial respiration. Transport to the veterinarian immediately and continue artificial respiration on the way to the veterinarian or until cat is breathing without assistance.

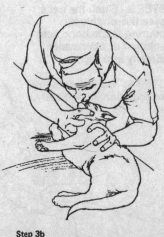

Step 3b

STEP 4: If the heart is not beating, perform CPR (cardiopulmonary resuscitation).

a. Turn the cat on its side.

b. Kneel down at the head of the cat.

c. Grasp the chest so that the breastbone is resting in the palm of your hand, your thumb on one side of the chest and your fingers on the other. Your thumb and fingers should fall about in the middle of the chest.

d. Compress the chest by firmly squeezing your thumb and fingers together for a count of "two" and release for a count of "one." Repeat about 30 times in 30 seconds.

e. Alternately (after 30 seconds), hold the cat's mouth and lips closed and blow firmly into its nostrils. Blow for three seconds, take a deep breath, and repeat until you feel resistance or see the chest rise. Try to repeat this 20 times in 60 seconds.

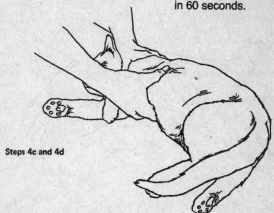

Steps 4c and 4d

continued

f. After one minute, stop. Look at the chest for breathing movement and feel for heartbeat by placing fingers about one inch behind the cat's elbow and in the center of its chest.

g. If the cat's heart is still not beating, continue CPR. If the heart starts beating, but the cat is still not breathing, return to Step 3b to continue artificial respiration.

STEP 5: Transport to the veterinarian immediately. CPR or artificial respiration should be continued on the way to the veterinarian or until the cat is breathing and its heart is beating without assistance.

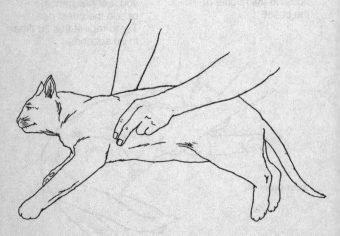

Step 4f

Toad Poisoning

SIGNS: EXCESSIVE DROOLING, SHAKING HEAD, TREMBLING AND SHAKING BODY, LACK OF COORDINATION, DIFFICULTY IN BREATHING, CONVULSIONS, COMA.

WATCH FOR SIGNS OF SHOCK:

Pale or white gums, rapid heartbeat and breathing. If signs are present see page 118.

STEP 1: Approach the cat (see page 7); then restrain if necessary (see page 8 or 13).

STEP 2: Flush the cat's mouth thoroughly with water, being careful not to choke it. Keep its head tilted at a slight downward angle.

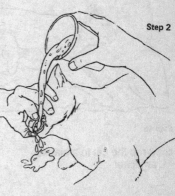

Step 2

Signs develop immediately after contact of the toad (Bufo species) with the mouth or eyes of the cat.

continued

STEP 3: Flush the cat's eyes thoroughly by pouring plain water directly into them.

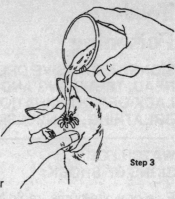

Step 3

STEP 4: If the cat is unconscious:

a. Move the cat onto a blanket, towel, or jacket.

b. Place a hot water bottle or container (100°F/37°C) against the cat's abdomen. Wrap the bottle in cloth to prevent burns.

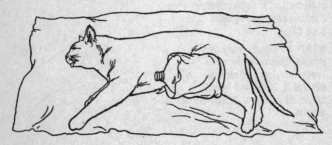

Step 4b

c. Wrap the cat in a blanket or jacket.

STEP 5: Transport to the veterinarian immediately.

Puncture Wound

SIGNS: BLOOD-TINGED FUR, LIMPING.

WATCH FOR SIGNS OF SHOCK:

Pale or white gums, rapid heartbeat and breathing. If signs are present see page 118.

A. If object (knife, arrow, stick, etc.) is protruding

STEP 1: Approach the cat (see page 7); then restrain if necessary (see page 8 or 13). Take care not to touch the object.

STEP 2: DO NOT attempt to remove the object.

STEP 3: Place clean cloths, sterile dressings, or sanitary napkins around the point of entry.

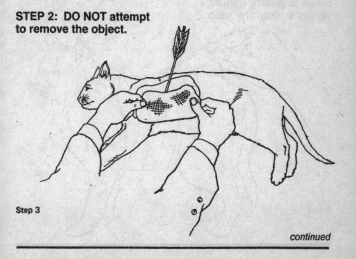

Step 3

continued

STEP 4: If the wound is in the chest, bandage tightly around the point of entry.

STEP 5: Transport immediately to the veterinarian.

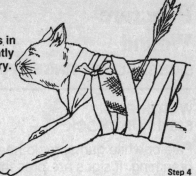

Step 4

B. Other puncture wounds

STEP 1: Approach the cat (see page 7); then restrain if necessary (see page 8 or 13).

STEP 2: If the wound is in the chest and a "sucking" noise is heard, bandage tightly enough to keep

air from entering and transport immediately to the veterinarian. If not, proceed to Step 3.

STEP 3: Clip the hair around the wound.

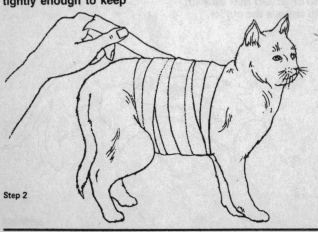

Step 2

STEP 4: Examine the wound carefully for foreign objects such as glass or wood splinters. If present, remove with tweezers or needle-nose pliers.

Step 4

STEP 5: Flush thoroughly by pouring 3% hydrogen peroxide into the wound. DO NOT use any other antiseptic.

Step 5

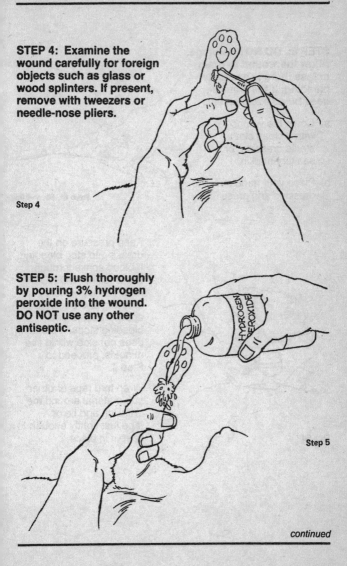

continued

**STEP 6: DO NOT bandage.
Allow the wound to drain
unless there is excessive
bleeding. If the wound
does bleed excessively:**

a. Cover the wound
with a clean cloth,
sterile dressing, or
sanitary napkin.

b. Place your hand over the
dressing and press firmly.

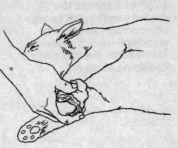

Steps 6a, 6b, and 6c

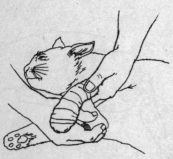

c. Keep pressure on the
dressing to stop bleeding.
If blood soaks through
the dressing, DO NOT
remove. Apply more
dressing and continue to
apply pressure until
bleeding stops. If bleeding
does not stop within five
minutes, proceed to
Step 7.

d. Wrap torn rags or other
soft material around the
dressing and tie or
tape just tightly enough to
keep it in place.

Step 6d

STEP 7: If bleeding does not stop within five minutes, apply a tourniquet. DO NOT apply a tourniquet to the head or torso.

Steps 7b and 7c

a. Use a tie or piece of cloth folded to about one inch width. DO NOT use rope, wire, or string.

b. Place the material between the wound and the heart, an inch or two above, but not touching, the wound.

c. Wrap the tie or cloth twice around the appendage and cross the ends.

d. Tie a stick or ruler to the material with a single knot.

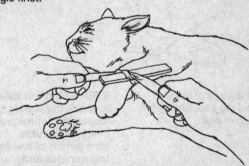

Step 7d

continued

e. Twist the stick
   until bleeding stops,
   but no tighter.

Step 7e

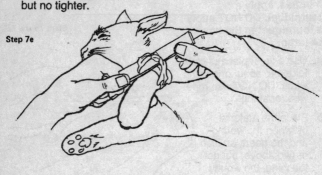

Step 7f

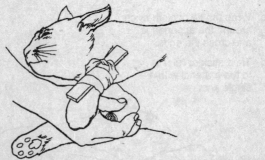

f. Wrap a piece of cloth
   around the stick and limb
   to keep in place.

**STEP 8: If it will take time
to reach the veterinarian,
loosen the tourniquet
every 15 minutes
for a period of one to
two minutes and
then retighten.**

**STEP 9: Transport to the
veterinarian immediately.**

Queening Problems

Any of the following requires immediate veterinary care:

a. Failure to deliver within three hours of intermittent labor.

b. Failure to deliver within 30 minutes of continuous hard labor.

c. Heavy bright red bleeding during labor.

d. Brown or foul-smelling discharge during labor.

e. General weakness of the mother.

f. Failure to deliver by the 66th day of gestation.

g. Presentation of the first water sac with no delivery after one hour.

A. If the kitten is stuck in the birth canal with half of its body exposed

STEP 1: Grasp the kitten with a clean towel.

It is absolutely vital to provide a secluded place for the mother to have her litter. After delivery, the kittens should not be touched or disturbed.

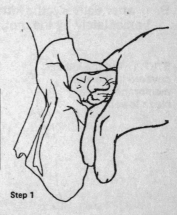

Step 1

continued

STEP 2: Applying steady traction, gently pull the kitten at a slight downward angle. Continue pulling gently and steadily until the kitten is delivered.

STEP 3: If you are unable to remove the kitten, or if the mother is uncooperative, contact the veterinarian immediately.

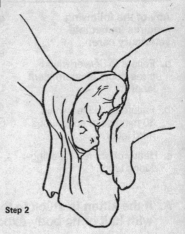

Step 2

B. If, after delivery, the kitten is not cleaned immediately by the mother

STEP 1: Put the kitten, covered in the fetal membrane, into a clean towel.

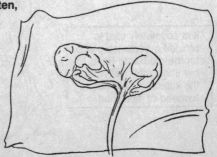

Step 1

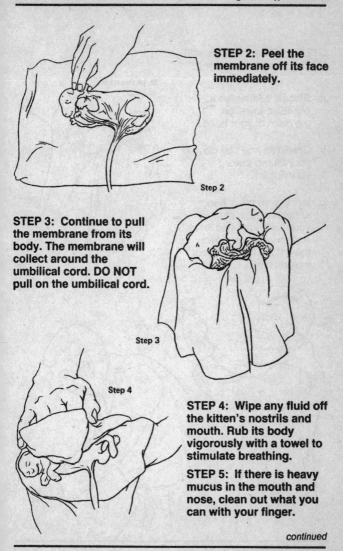

STEP 2: Peel the membrane off its face immediately.

Step 2

STEP 3: Continue to pull the membrane from its body. The membrane will collect around the umbilical cord. DO NOT pull on the umbilical cord.

Step 3

Step 4

STEP 4: Wipe any fluid off the kitten's nostrils and mouth. Rub its body vigorously with a towel to stimulate breathing.

STEP 5: If there is heavy mucus in the mouth and nose, clean out what you can with your finger.

continued

STEP 6: If the kitten is still having trouble breathing:

Steps 6a and 6b

a. Place the kitten on its back in a towel on the palm of your hand.

b. Cradle its head by closing your thumb toward your fingers.

c. Using your other hand to secure the kitten, lift your hands to head level and swing firmly down toward the floor. Repeat several times.

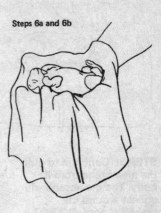

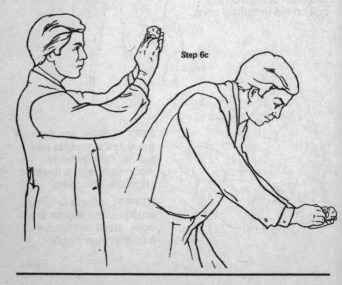

Step 6c

d. Vigorously rub the kitten
   again with the towel.

e. Stop when the kitten
   is actively moving
   and crying. Step 6d

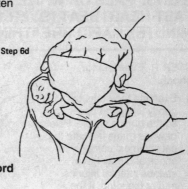

**STEP 7: Tie a thread
around the umbilical cord
about one inch above
the kitten's abdomen.
Leaving the tied portion
attached to the kitten, cut
off the rest of the umbilical
cord and fetal membrane.**

**STEP 8: Place the kitten
with its mother. She will
take care of the rest. If she
does not take care of the
kittens, or if any other
problem develops, contact
the veterinarian as soon
as possible.**

Step 7

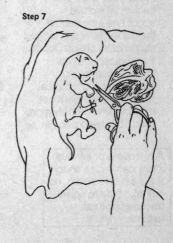

Shock

SIGNS: PALE OR WHITE GUMS, VERY FAST HEARTBEAT (OVER 150 BEATS PER MINUTE), RAPID BREATHING.

STEP 1: Examine for shock.

Step 1a

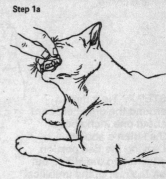

a. Examine the gums by gently lifting the upper lip so the gum is visible. Pale or white gums indicate the cat is almost certainly in shock and may have serious internal injuries and/or bleeding. If the gums are pink the cat is probably not in shock.

b. Determine the heartbeat. Place your fingers firmly on the cat's chest about one inch behind the cat's elbow and in the center of its chest. Count the number of beats in ten seconds and multiply by six. If the cat is in shock its heartbeat may be considerably more than 150 beats per minute.

Step 1b

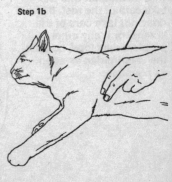

> Any trauma or serious injury can cause shock. If the cat is in shock, do not take time to splint fractures or treat minor injuries.

STEP 2: Place the cat on a blanket, towel, or jacket on its side with its head extended.

STEP 3: Clear the airway.

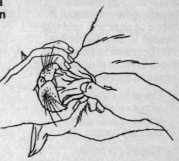

a. Place one hand over the cat's head so that your thumb and index finger fall just behind the long canines (fang teeth), the head resting against your palm.

b. Gently tilt the cat's head back so its nose is pointing upward. Push your thumb toward your finger; the mouth will open.

Steps 3a, 3b, and 3c

c. Gently pull out the cat's tongue to keep the airway open. If the cat resists your attempt to pull the tongue out, do not repeat Step 3.

STEP 4: Elevate the cat's hindquarters slightly by placing them on a pillow or folded or rolled up towel.

Step 4

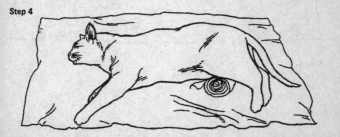

continued

STEP 5: Stop visible bleeding immediately; if blood is spurting and the wound is on a leg or the tail, proceed to Step 6. If there is no visible bleeding proceed to Step 8.

a. Cover the wound with a clean cloth, sterile dressing, or sanitary napkin.

b. Place your hand over the dressing and press firmly.

c. Keep pressure on the dressing to stop bleeding. If blood soaks through the dressing, DO NOT remove. Apply more dressing and continue to apply pressure until bleeding stops. If bleeding does not stop within five minutes, proceed to Step 6.

d. Wrap rags or other soft material around the dressing and tie or tape just tightly enough to keep it in place.

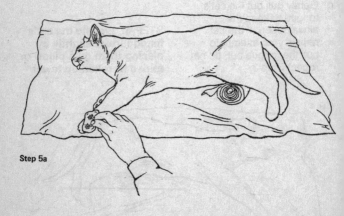

Step 5a

STEP 6: Apply a tourniquet.

a. Use a tie or piece of cloth folded to about one inch width. DO NOT use rope, wire, or string.

b. Place the material between the wound and the heart, an inch or two above, but not touching, the wound.

c. Wrap the tie or cloth twice around the appendage and cross the ends.

d. Tie a stick or ruler to the material with a single knot.

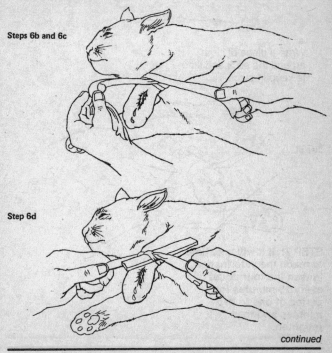

Steps 6b and 6c

Step 6d

continued

e. Twist the stick until
   bleeding stops,
   but no tighter.

Step 6e

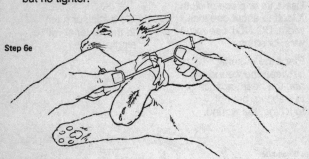

f. Wrap a piece of cloth
   around the stick and limb
   to keep in place.

Step 6f

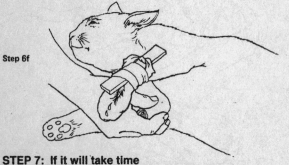

**STEP 7: If it will take time
to reach the veterinarian,
loosen the tourniquet
every 15 minutes for a
period of one to two
minutes and then
retighten.**

STEP 8: Conserve body heat.

a. Place a hot water bottle or container (100°F/37°C) against the cat's abdomen. Wrap the bottle in cloth to prevent burns.

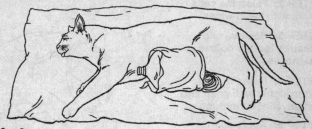

Step 8a

b. Wrap the cat in a blanket or jacket.

STEP 9: Transport to the veterinarian immediately.

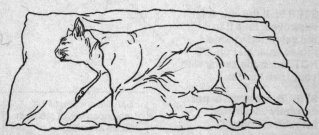

Step 8b

Skunk Encounter

STEP 1: Approach the cat (see page 7); then restrain if necessary (see page 8 or 13).

STEP 2: Flush the cat's eyes with fresh water.

STEP 3: Remove and destroy leather collars or harnesses.

STEP 4: Bathe the cat thoroughly with soap and water. Rinse thoroughly.

STEP 5: Apply plain tomato juice liberally. After several minutes, bathe again with soap and water. Time will eventually remove the odor. Skunk odor neutralizers are available.

STEP 6: If the skunk is destroyed, take it to the veterinarian for a rabies examination. DO NOT touch the skunk with your bare hands.

STEP 7: If the cat is not currently vaccinated for rabies, contact the veterinarian.

Step 2

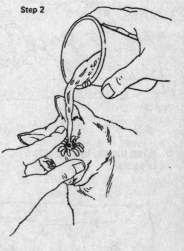

Skunks are one of the major carriers of rabies in North America.

Poisonous Snakebite

SIGNS: TWO FANG MARKS, PAIN, SWELLING, VOMITING, DIFFICULTY IN BREATHING, POSSIBLE PARALYSIS AND CONVULSIONS.

WATCH FOR SIGNS OF SHOCK:

Pale or white gums, rapid heartbeat and breathing. If signs are present see page 118.

Treatment must begin as soon as possible after the bite. If possible, kill the snake so it can be taken to the veterinarian. Otherwise, try to remember identifying marks.

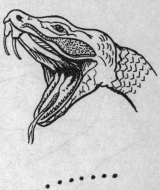

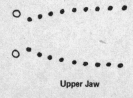

Upper Jaw

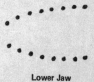

Lower Jaw

continued

STEP 1: Approach the cat (see page 7); then restrain if necessary (see page 8 or 13).

STEP 2: If the bite is on the head or torso, proceed to Step 3. If the bite is on a leg or the tail, apply a tourniquet.

a. Use a tie or piece of cloth folded to about one inch wide. DO NOT use rope, wire, or string.

b. Place the material between the bite and the heart, an inch or two above, but not touching, the bite.

c. Wrap the tie or cloth twice around the appendage and cross the ends.

Steps 2b and 2c

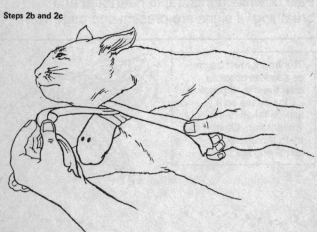

d. Tie a stick or ruler
   to the material with a
   single knot.

Step 2d

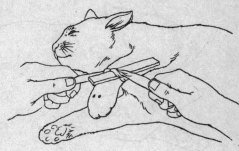

e. Twist the stick just
   tightly enough to cut
   off circulation to
   the bite area.

Step 2e

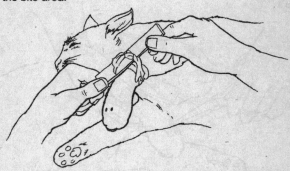

continued

127

f. Wrap a piece of cloth
   around the stick and limb
   to keep in place.

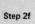

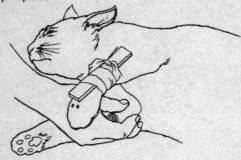

STEP 3: Clip the hair from the bite area.

Step 3

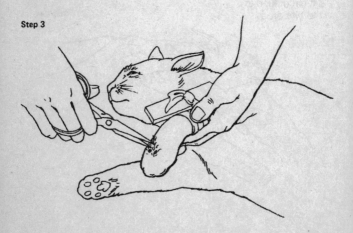

STEP 4: Make a single cut over each fang mark with a knife, just deep enough to draw blood.

Step 4

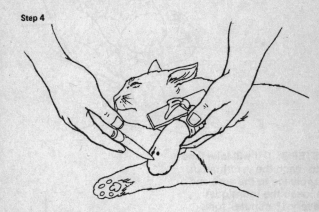

STEP 5: Use your mouth to suck venom from the bite. Use heavy suction and repeat several times. Spit out the blood, DO NOT swallow it.

Step 5

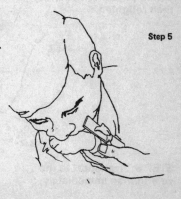

CAUTION: Do not use this technique if you have open sores or cuts on your lips, tongue, or inside cheeks; the poison can be absorbed into your system.

continued

129

STEP 6: Flush thoroughly by pouring 3% hydrogen peroxide directly on the bite. DO NOT use any other antiseptic.

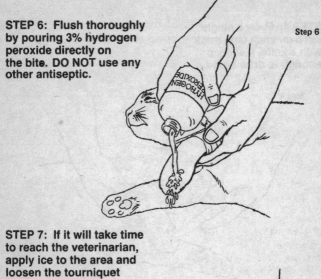

Step 6

STEP 7: If it will take time to reach the veterinarian, apply ice to the area and loosen the tourniquet every 15 minutes for a period of just 10 seconds, then retighten.

Step 7

STEP 8: Transport to the veterinarian immediately.

Nonpoisonous Snakebite

SIGNS: "U"-SHAPED BITE, PAIN IN BITE AREA.

If possible, kill the snake so it can be taken to the veterinarian. Otherwise, try to remember identifying marks.

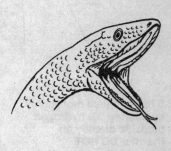

STEP 1: If you are not certain snake is nonpoisonous, and you cannot get to a veterinarian immediately, treat as a poisonous snake bite. See page 125.

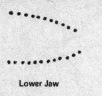

Lower Jaw

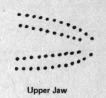

Upper Jaw

STEP 2: Approach the cat (see page 7); then restrain if necessary (see page 8 or 13).

continued

STEP 3: Clip the hair from the bite area.

Step 3

STEP 4: Flush thoroughly by pouring 3% hydrogen peroxide directly on the bite. DO NOT use any other antiseptic.

Step 4

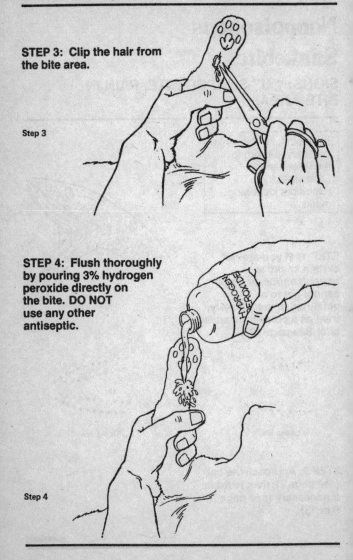

Swallowing Thread, String, or Yarn

SIGNS: THREAD, STRING, OR YARN HANGING OUT OF THE MOUTH OR RECTUM; VOMITING COMBINED WITH HISTORY OF PLAYING WITH THREAD, STRING, OR YARN; LOSS OF APPETITE WITH ABOVE SIGNS.

STEP 1: Approach the cat (see page 7); then restrain if necessary (see page 8 or 13).

STEP 2: If nothing is visible, proceed to Step 3. If thread, string, or yarn is hanging out of the cat's mouth or rectum:

a. Pull lightly. If you feel resistance, stop. DO NOT continue to pull.

b. Cut off as short as possible and proceed to Step 3.

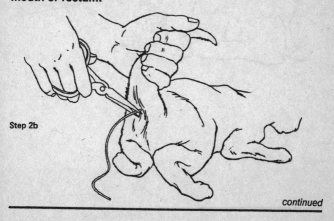

Step 2b

continued

STEP 3: Give the cat one tablespoon of white petroleum jelly. Using a small amount each time, rub the jelly on the cat's mouth and paws. The cat will lick it off. DO NOT give mineral oil.

STEP 4: If vomiting occurs or the cat stops eating, transport to the veterinarian immediately.

Step 3

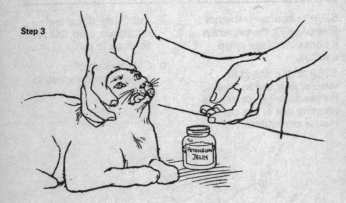

Unconsciousness

STEP 1: If you suspect choking, see page 59.

STEP 2: If the cat is breathing, check for shock. See page 118. If the cat is not breathing, proceed to Step 3.

STEP 3: Feel for heartbeat by placing fingers about one inch behind the cat's elbow and in the center of its chest.

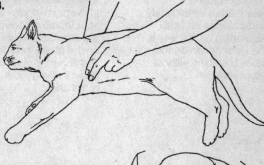

Step 3

STEP 4: If the heart is not beating, proceed to Step 5. If it is beating, perform artificial respiration.

a. Turn the cat on its side.

b. Hold the cat's mouth and lips closed and blow firmly into its nostrils. Blow for three seconds, take a deep breath, and repeat until you feel resistance or see the chest rise.

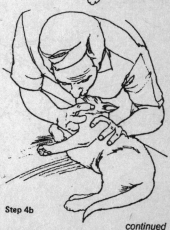

Step 4b

continued

c. After one minute, stop. Watch the chest for movement to indicate the cat is breathing on its own.

d. If the cat is still not breathing, continue artificial respiration.

e. Transport to the veterinarian immediately and continue artificial respiration on the way to the veterinarian or until cat is breathing without assistance.

STEP 5: If the heart is not beating, perform CPR (cardiopulmonary resuscitation).

a. Turn the cat on its side.

b. Kneel down at the head of the cat.

c. Grasp the chest so that the breastbone is resting in the palm of your hand, your thumb on one side of the chest and your fingers on the other. Your thumb and fingers should fall about in the middle of the chest.

Steps 5c and 5d

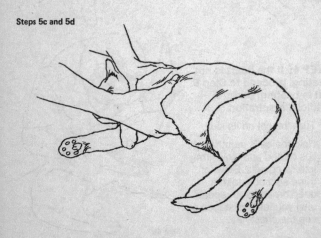

d. Compress the chest by firmly squeezing your thumb and fingers together for a count of "two" and release for a count of "one." Repeat about 30 times in 30 seconds.

e. Alternately (after 30 seconds), hold the cat's mouth and lips closed and blow firmly into its nostrils. Blow for three seconds, take a deep breath, and repeat until you feel resistance or see the chest rise. Try to repeat this 20 times in 60 seconds.

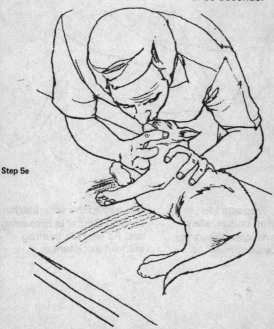

Step 5e

continued

f. After one minute, stop. Look at the chest for breathing movement and feel for heartbeat by placing fingers about one inch behind the cat's elbow and in the center of its chest.

g. If the cat's heart is still not beating, continue CPR. If the heart starts beating, but the cat is still not breathing, return to Step 4b to continue artificial respiration.

Step 5f

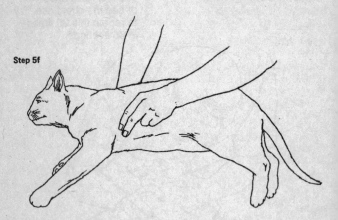

STEP 6: Transport to the veterinarian immediately. CPR or artificial respiration should be continued on the way to the veterinarian or until the cat is breathing and its heart is beating without assistance.

Vomiting

STEP 1: Remove all food and water immediately.

STEP 2: If vomiting contains blood or is frequent, contact the veterinarian immediately. If not, proceed to Step 3.

STEP 3: Treat with Pepto-Bismol® every four hours at the rate of ½ teaspoons per five to seven pounds of the cat's weight.
See Administering Oral Medicine, page 19.

STEP 4: DO NOT attempt to feed or give water for at least 12 hours.

STEP 5: After 12 hours, feed the cat a mixture of small quantities of steamed ground beef, cooked rice, and cottage cheese. If the cat rejects the ground beef, substitute boiled chicken breasts, skinned and boned. If this is held down, a transition to regular diet should take place over the next two days by mixing an increasing quantity of regular cat food with the ground beef or chicken mix.

The Whys of Emergency Treatment

Approaching an Injured Cat

To successfully help an injured cat, you must remember it has five weapons—the mouth and four sets of claws. It is discouraging to be scratched or bitten by a frightened pet you are trying to assist. But because it is frightened, it will either run or, if cornered, attack.

Therefore, when approaching an injured cat, move slowly and talk reassuringly. Stoop down to the cat's level so it feels more comfortable with your presence. Watch the eyes and body language to see the cat's reaction to you. If the cat is shivering and crouching, you can attempt to pet it for reassurance. Pet the cat behind the head first. If it lets you pet it in this area, then pet the rest of the head and neck area.

Scratching the ears and stroking under the chin are very comforting to a cat; it will often push its head up into your hand for more of this attention. However, if the cat is hissing, growling, and striking out with its paws, it may be very difficult to handle. Some cats react this way for only a short time to test your patience. It is a good idea to continue to talk to the cat for a few minutes to see if it will calm down enough for you to be able to restrain it.

Restraining an Injured Cat

Once you have approached the cat and determined if it is cooperative or uncooperative, the next step is to choose the method of restraint that will best fit the circumstances. Your choice will depend upon the availability of an assistant, the type and location of the cat's injury, and the first aid treatment necessary.

Restraining a cooperative cat means keeping it still so that treatment can be administered properly. The lifting procedure is easy as long as you avoid fumbling and use quick, decisive movements. Prepare for situations that need quick and thoughtful action by familiarizing yourself with the proper techniques shown on pages 8-12. Some cats prefer to be held in your arms during treatment; others will need to be restrained on a table. When restraining on a table, try to select a surface with which the cat is unfamiliar. This puts the cat in a precarious situation, which may help keep it cautious and subdued.

When the cat is uncooperative, the restraint is used not only to quiet the cat so that first aid can be administered, but also to protect you from injury. Again, the cat's weapons are its mouth and claws.

The best way to handle an uncooperative cat is to drop a blanket or towel over it and scoop it up quickly. Be sure all four paws are inside the cover. Then, the injured portion of the body can be exposed for treatment, or the cat can be transported to the veterinarian.

Some cats are impossible to handle when injured. In this case, drop the blanket or towel over the cat and gather the edges together to form a bag. As a rule, a cat feels secure covered or in a box. It may struggle a little, but you are protected. Once at the veterinarian's office, he or she can tranquilize the cat before treatment.

Transporting an Injured Cat

The injured cat can be transported to the veterinarian either held in your arms or placed in a cardboard box or cat carrier. If you suspect a broken back, try not to move the cat more than necessary to avoid further injury to the spinal cord. Tie the cat gently onto a stiff board to prevent movement while being transported to the veterinarian, and have someone call ahead to be certain he or she is prepared for your arrival.

Abscess

An abscess is a localized infection filled with pus. The body creates walls around these wounds and the pus collects within the confines of the walls.

Abscesses in cats are usually caused by bite wounds or scratches, and may be multiple when they occur. The infection results from bacteria carried on the teeth or claws of the attacking animal, which enters the skin through the bite or scratch. Most abscesses will be located around the neck, front legs, or the tail and rump area. Many times owners fail to realize the cat has been bitten until they find a soft painful swelling on the body or a foul-smelling discharge on the fur.

Fur should be clipped from the suspected area to make cleaning easier and also to aid in drainage of the wound. The area should then be flushed thoroughly with 3% hydrogen peroxide if the abscess is open. If the abscess has not yet broken open, hot compresses should be applied for 20 minutes two or three times per day until it opens and starts draining. Never try to cut an abscess open yourself to establish drainage. This should be left to a veterinarian. The cat may lick the abscess in an attempt to open it if the affected area is within its reach. When it does open, 3% hydrogen peroxide should be used liberally to help kill the bacteria. If the abscess is discovered too late, there may be extensive damage to the muscles and other tissues under the skin. This requires professional attention as soon as possible. It is advisable to keep a draining abscess open for two or three days by picking the scab off. This will prevent buildup of the pus and speed healing.

Animal Bite

If your cat has been in a fight, examine it carefully for hidden wounds. You'll often find punctures around the neck area, rump area, and on the legs. Look through the hair carefully to find blood stains, which would indicate the skin has been punctured.

After clipping the hair from around the wound to assess the damage, flush with 3% hydrogen peroxide to prevent infection. This is one of the major complications of a bite.

Although there may be only a few punctures, extensive damage may have been done to underlying muscles. If the wounds are deep enough to require stitches, this should be done as soon as possible by a professional.

Unless there is extensive bleeding, the wounds should be left open to drain until the cat is seen by the veterinarian. Whenever tissue is damaged, fluid accumulates in the area. If the wound is not left open to drain, a painful swelling will occur and the site will become a perfect medium for the growth of bacteria and infection.

If possible, it is important to determine if the biting animal has been inoculated against rabies. If the biting animal is a wild animal such as a skunk or raccoon, efforts should be made to destroy it so the brain can be examined for rabies. Never touch the animal with your bare hands, even after it has been killed. Wear gloves or wrap the body in a blanket. Your veterinarian will take care of the rabies examination.

Bladder Infection

An area of concern to cat owners and veterinarians is bladder infections, medically known as Feline Urological Syndrome or cystitis. This disease is not limited to male cats, but is of great danger to them because of their anatomy. The male cat has an extremely small tube (urethra) leading from the bladder through the penis. In most cases cystitis causes the formation of a crystalline substance in the urine, which will clog the urethra of male cats and make urination impossible. This will be evidenced by the cat straining in the litter pan as if constipated and producing only small drops of urine, crying while straining, squatting outside the litter pan, and licking its genital area frequently. If the cat is plugged and cannot urinate, the kidneys will lose the ability to remove the waste products from the blood. This causes a buildup of nitrogen by-products in the blood known as uremia, which can lead to death. A blocked male cat that is vomiting is probably uremic and will die if not treated immediately. Call your veterinarian, regardless of the time of day or night.

Female cats also get cystitis, and though the symptoms are the same as those of a male, females will not plug up, and the midnight emergency does not exist.

Many causes of cystitis have been suggested; virus and diet are two. Researchers are working to find the definitive cause. As yet, we have many theories but no answers.

At the present time veterinarians are recommending a low ash diet in order to decrease mineral intake, thus possibly preventing crystal formation in the urine. They also suggest making sure the cat drinks plenty of water. Several surgical procedures have been developed to help prevent obstruction in the male. While these procedures are very successful, the cat can still have uncomfortable attacks of cystitis.

Bleeding

With a bleeding injury, the main purpose of first aid is to prevent excessive blood loss that can lead to shock. Pressure applied to the wound allows the normal clotting mechanism of the blood to stop the leak. This is a complex process, but basically the blood cells form a fine screen over the wound and thus prevent further loss of blood. That is why it is important not to remove the dressing once it has been applied. If you lift it to look at the wound, it will break up the clots that are forming and the wound will continue to bleed.

If the wound continues to bleed through the dressing, it will be necessary to use a tourniquet. The tourniquet should be used only as a last resort, because although it stops the bleeding, it also prevents blood from getting to other tissues in the area, which become oxygen starved and die.

Blood is carried from the heart by the arteries and returned by the veins. If an artery is cut, the blood will spurt with each beat of the heart. Cut arteries require immediate care to stop the bleeding and usually require veterinary care for repair.

Internal bleeding can be caused by a ruptured liver or spleen as the result of an accident, or the ingestion of an anticoagulant such as rat or mouse poison. Symptoms are pale or white gums; rapid heartbeat and breathing; availability of rat or mouse poison; and bleeding from the ears, nose, or mouth with any of the above signs. Shock almost always follows. Therefore, the cat's tongue should be gently pulled forward to keep the airway open, and the hindquarters should be elevated slightly. It is important to conserve body heat by placing a wrapped hot water bottle against the abdomen and wrapping the cat in a blanket or jacket. Since shock is often fatal, transport the cat to the veterinarian immediately.

An injured ear will bleed heavily because the skin over the ear is so thin. Cats' ears will usually stop bleeding within five minutes after pressure is applied, unless the ear is severely cut. Veterinary attention should then be sought to repair these injuries to keep the proper shape of the ear.

Cats love to keep their nails sharp. Often, their nails will break during a fight or because they are too long. There is a blood vessel and nerve in the center of each nail. This is seen as the pink area in white nails. If you cut your cat's nails yourself, it is important not to cut into the "quick," as it is called, but to clip the nail just in front of it. If the "quick" is cut, the nail will bleed and the cut nerve will cause some pain. If your cat is nervous or upset, have a professional cut its nails.

Bleeding from the nose is rare in cats. It is usually due to external trauma such as automobile accidents, falls from a great height, or fights. Ice packs applied to the cat's nose will constrict the blood vessels and allow clotting to take place. If bleeding continues, this may indicate a serious disorder, and immediate veterinary attention is required.

Broken Bones

With cats, as with human beings, all bones are subject to breakage, but leg fractures are by far the most common. It is important to remember that cats have a high pain tolerance, and often a dangling leg seems to cause no pain. Therefore, don't be afraid to handle the fractured limb (gently!). The cat will let you know if it hurts. If the cat is in pain or if the fracture is open, do not attempt to splint. An open fracture is one in which the bone protrudes or there is a break in the skin over the broken bone. First aid efforts should be directed to the control of infection, since the exposed bone is subject to bacterial invasion. Proper cleaning is of prime importance. Use only 3% hydrogen peroxide, as other antiseptics may cause tissue damage. Then, hold a large towel under the limb for support and transport the cat to the veterinarian.

A closed fracture is one with the bone broken but the skin intact. The leg should be splinted, but do not confuse splinting with setting the limb. The limb should be set by a professional. Splinting is only a temporary procedure, so you may use any firm material at hand. The purpose of a splint is to prevent further damage by immobilizing the limb, and to make the animal more comfortable during the trip.

In severe accidents, spinal or rib fractures can occur. If the cat is paralyzed, or if there is an unusual arch to the back, the back may be broken. To prevent further damage to the spinal cord, it is very important that you do not move the cat more than necessary. The spinal cord lies inside the bony vertebrae of the back. If these vertebrae are bent while moving the cat, more severe damage can occur to the irreparable spinal cord. It is for this reason that the utmost care must be taken while sliding the cat onto a flat board for transportation.

Broken ribs are not quite as frequent in cats as in dogs. When they do occur, it is important to take care in handling the cat. Occasionally, a fractured rib will enter the thorax (chest cavity) and the sharp bone can puncture a lung or even the heart. If the cat can be handled, bandage the chest to prevent further damage. However, if the cat is uncontrollable, do not attempt bandaging. Simply wrap it in a blanket and transport it to the veterinarian.

Burns

Burns can be caused by fire, heat, boiling liquids, chemicals, and electricity. All are painful and can cause damage, even death. Most scalds can be avoided by care in the kitchen. Because the cat is often on countertops or underfoot while its owner is cooking, care should be taken when handling hot water or cooking oil.

Superficial burns, evidenced by pain and reddening of the skin, are usually not serious. However, first aid should be given as soon as possible to ease the pain. Burns tend to "cook" the skin, and in order to stop this "cooking" process, cold water or ice packs should be applied at once to the burned area.

At one time, the recommended treatment was the application of butter or grease, until it was discovered that these products could actually make the wound worse. They should never be used.

Third degree burns are far more serious. Depending on how much of the body is involved, they can cause death. The deeper the layers of skin involved, the more likely the cat is to go into shock. The outer skin layers are destroyed, and the unprotected lower layers are then susceptible to infection. If the burns are extensive, a great deal of fluid from the tissue cells will be lost and shock is certain to result. Treatment for shock is your first priority and should be continued until professional help can be obtained.

In burns due to fire, the airway and lungs may also be seriously damaged by inhalation of smoke and heated air. Burned lungs collect fluid, causing shortness of breath. To ease breathing, the cat's head should be kept higher than its body. Also, a burned airway may swell shut; it is imperative to keep this airway open. Immediate professional help is essential.

Chemical burns can also endanger our pets. Products such as drain cleaners or paint thinner can cause serious skin damage, and poisoning if swallowed. To prevent accidents of this nature, these products should be kept out of the cat's reach.

If you notice a chemical odor on your cat, often the first sign of this type of burn, bathe it immediately. Do not use solvents of any kind on the skin. Use mild soap, lather well, then rinse thoroughly until the odor has disappeared.

Unlike with heat burns, a soothing antibiotic ointment can be applied to the affected area until the cat can be seen by a veterinarian. Be sure all the chemical is removed before the ointment is applied.

Choking

When a cat is choking on a foreign object, it needs help at once. The harder it tries to breathe, the more panicky it becomes. Your goal is to open the airway without being bitten. If you cannot reach the object with your fingers or needle-nose pliers, or if the cat is struggling too much to let you try, turn it upside down and shake it. This will often dislodge the object and propel it out of the mouth.

Another method that may be used is similar to the Heimlich maneuver in humans. This abdominal compression technique can be compared to pushing the air out of a beach ball. Sudden thrusts on the abdomen cause the diaphragm to bulge forward into the chest. This, in turn, forces air, and frequently the object, out of the windpipe.

If the animal is unconscious and you believe a foreign object is present, you must open the airway before giving artificial respiration or cardiac massage. If the cat cannot breathe, efforts to revive it will be fruitless.

The method of artificial respiration presented in this book is the most effective. Blowing directly into the cat's nostrils fully inflates the lungs and the result is maximum oxygenation of the blood.

Cardiac massage keeps the blood pumping through the vessels and stimulates the heart muscle to contract and start beating again. With cats, you compress the heart by actually squeezing it between your thumb and fingers. This helps keep the blood pressure up and hopefully will start normal heart muscle contractions. If the brain becomes blood starved and receives no oxygen, death will follow. If you are in doubt about how long you should continue CPR, keep doing it until you see the cat breathing by itself or until you can get to a veterinarian. You can never overdo CPR, and continued efforts may actually save a life.

Convulsion/Seizure

A convulsion or seizure is rarely fatal, but it is a frightening experience when seen for the first time. It is the result of constant electrical firing from the brain to the muscles of the body.

It is important not to panic. You are not in danger, but the cat needs help to protect it from self-injury. Pull it away from walls and furniture and, if possible, wrap it in a blanket or towel. Do not attempt to place anything in its mouth. This will not help, and you may be bitten. The cat is not aware of its actions during the seizure, which usually lasts only a few minutes. This is followed by 15 minutes to a half hour of recovery time, during which period the cat may be dazed and confused.

Not all seizures are due to simple epilepsy, which is, in fact, rare in cats. Most seizures are due to toxic substances, brain tumors, liver disease, parasites, or viral diseases. Seizures or convulsions should never be taken lightly. The problem should be discussed with a veterinarian as soon as possible.

Diarrhea

D iarrhea is a commonly encountered problem that occurs when food is passed through the intestine too rapidly. It can be caused by allergies, milk, worms, spoiled food, or plants. There are also more serious causes such as tumors, viral infections, and diseases of the liver, pancreas, and kidney.

Initial treatment at home should be conservative, with a diet that is bland, easily digested, and binding. Follow the steps on page 66. However, it is important to seek professional help if signs of blood, severe depression, or abdominal pain are present.

Drowning

C ats are naturally adequate swimmers for short distances, but they can get into trouble. Sometimes they get too far from the shore and tire trying to swim back, or fall into a swimming pool and cannot get up the steep sides.

Always protect yourself when trying to rescue a drowning cat. A few extra moments of preparation can save two lives, yours and the cat's. Once the cat is on land, you must first get the water out of its lungs. To do this, the cat can simply be lifted by the hind legs, turned upside down, and shaken vigorously. Failure to eliminate this water will certainly lead to death.

When the lungs have been cleared, if the cat is unconscious, it is important to check for a heartbeat and breathing. If necessary, perform cardiopulmonary resuscitation (CPR). Many cats that appear to be dead can be revived with CPR; but if the water has not been drained from the lungs first, your efforts will be useless.

Electrical Shock

G rown cats are seldom victims of electrical shock. But kittens are naturally curious and will chew almost anything, including electric cords. If the insulation is punctured and the mouth comes in contact with both wires, the cat will receive a shock and may be unable to release the cord.

You must disconnect the cord from the socket immediately, before touching the cat. If you touch the cat before disconnecting the cord, you can also be electrocuted.

Once the cord is disconnected, you can safely touch the cat. Examine it carefully. Electrocution can cause severe heart damage and fluid accumulation in the lungs. Strong shock can stop the heart, and cardiopulmonary resuscitation (CPR) must be performed immediately to start the heart beating again.

Often, the mouth will be burned from contact with the bare wires. This looks much more serious than it is, and will heal eventually if cleaned and treated properly.

Most electrical shocks require professional attention; the cat should be taken to the veterinarian as soon as possible.

Eye Injuries

I rritations to the eye can be caused by viruses, allergies, dust and dirt, fights, etc. An irritation can result in a mild inflammation of the tissue around the eye (conjunctivitis) or severe damage to the cornea. Upper respiratory diseases are probably the most common cause of conjunctivitis in cats.

When examining the eye, it is important to know that cats have a third eyelid located in the corner of the eye nearest the nose. This third eyelid can completely cover the eyeball and sometimes gives the appearance that part of the eye is gone. If it is raised and looks red, the eye is inflamed. Do not touch or manipulate this eyelid.

Other indications that the eye is irritated are squinting and rubbing or pawing at the eye. Your first priority is to prevent self-injury; this often causes more serious damage than the original irritation. Bandaging the dewclaw on the front paw of the affected side will help to prevent further damage from scratching. Placing a large piece of cardboard, shaped into an Elizabethan-type collar, around the cat's neck will prevent any scratching. All eye irritations should be treated by a veterinarian.

Fall from High-Rise Building

This problem is often referred to as High-Rise Syndrome, a colorful name coined by veterinarians who practice in areas where tall apartment buildings abound. Apartment cats frequently sit in a window and gaze at the birds as they fly by, or try to catch insects that land on the window sills. Unfortunately, not all windows are protected by sturdy screens, and occasionally the mesmerized cat springs at the bird or insect, and down it goes.

Veterinarians have found that a cat usually survives a fall of up to three stories without serious injury. In a fall from a greater height, the tendency to land on all four feet usually holds true and leg fractures are common. As the cat hits the ground, the head is thrust downward and the chin hits first. This usually breaks teeth and splits the upper palate, which causes the nose to bleed. Shock and internal injuries occur.

Frostbite

When a cat is exposed to freezing temperatures for a long period of time, there is always the possibility of frostbite. The areas most likely to be frostbitten are those that have little or no hair, and the ears and tail, which have a limited blood supply.

The affected areas should be warmed with moist heat, which will help to restore circulation. Frequently, the skin may turn very dark, which means the tissue is dead. If damage from frostbite is severe, part of the tail or ear tips may actually fall off. Frostbite should be treated by a professional immediately.

Hairball

Cats are fastidious, and this often causes a hairball problem. Cats groom themselves by licking their fur. The cat's tongue feels rather like sandpaper to the touch because of its many small barbs. These barbs catch the hair as the cat licks itself, and the hair is swallowed. If enough hair collects in the stomach without passing into the intestinal tract, the cat will vomit in an effort to rid itself of it. A successfully vomited hairball often looks like a long cigar. If there is more hair than can be brought up, the cat will vomit its food, because there is no room for it in the stomach. These cats act normally, are hungry, and may try to eat the vomited food.

Treatment is aimed at eliminating the hair from the stomach by coating the stomach so the hair will pass into the intestine and the stool. White petroleum jelly (Vaseline) is an excellent coating substance. Some cats like the taste and will lick it right off the spoon. It is also easily administered by placing one or two teaspoons on the mouth and paws; the cat will lick it off.

Treatment should be repeated daily until the petroleum jelly and hair are passed in the stool and the vomiting stops. It is important to realize that if the cat is depressed and not interested in food, or if the vomiting continues for more than two or three days, the problem is probably not hairballs. Veterinary attention should be sought as soon as possible.

Heart Muscle Disease

There are few diseases that cause a seemingly healthy cat to suddenly be on death's doorstep. Cardiomyopathy, or heart muscle disease, and subsequent aortic embolism (a clot in the artery) is one of them.

Cats that have certain forms of cardiomyopathy may simply not act right and a veterinarian will be able to discover the problem by electrocardiograms, radiographs, and listening to the cat's heart. Another form of heart muscle disease may go unnoticed until suddenly the cat loses function of the back legs, cries out as if in pain, and has difficulty breathing as evidenced by panting. The paralysis of the rear legs is due to a blood clot leaving the diseased heart, traveling down the major blood vessel (aorta) that supplies the body, and lodging at the division of the aorta to the vessels of the back legs. This cuts off the blood supply to the back legs and results in paralysis. The rear limbs of these cats will feel very cold to the touch in comparison to the rest of the body. Professional emergency treatment is needed to save the cat's life. Unfortunately, despite all efforts, most of these cats will die.

Veterinarians have no answers as to why cardiomyopathies occur, but research is continuing on this perplexing problem.

Heatstroke

Heatstroke is caused by the inability of the body to maintain its normal temperature because of environmental heat. It is often caused by keeping a cat in a hot area without adequate ventilation.

Prompt treatment is urgent. Body temperature often gets as high as 107°F/41.5°C, and without quick cooling severe brain damage and death will occur.

Your first goal is to cool the body by immersing the cat in a cold water bath or running a garden hose on the body; either treatment is to be continued for at least 30 minutes. Then apply ice packs to the head, and keep them in place while transporting the cat to a veterinarian.

Heatstroke can be prevented by making sure your cat has plenty of shade and ventilation. If you must take your cat driving with you, park in the shade and leave all the windows partially open.

Hypothermia

Exposure to either cold water or freezing temperatures can cause hypothermia, or subnormal body temperature. Survival will depend on how low the body temperature drops. A cat's normal body temperature is 100-101°F/38°C. If it drops below 90°F/32°C for any length of time, normal bodily functions will be severely impaired.

First aid treatment at home requires warming the cat with blankets, hot water bottles, or a heating pad. Hypothermia always requires veterinary attention as soon as these initial efforts to warm the cat have been made.

Insect Sting or Spider Bite

If a cat has been strung by a bee, wasp, yellow jacket, or hornet, the area quickly becomes swollen and somewhat painful. The raised area is called a wheal, and if the cat has been stung more than once, you will see several of these. A possible allergic reaction to the venom deposited by the insect is the most serious problem with this type of bite.

Stings and bites from certain arachnids including the brown recluse and black widow spiders, scorpions, and tarantulas are different. The pain is more intense and the wound heals more slowly, often with an open sore. There may be generalized reaction with vomiting and shivering. The vomiting is probably a mild allergic reaction, and the shivering is most likely due to generalized soreness. In any event, initial treatment is the same. That is, apply ice to the area and give a cold capsule containing an antihistamine. If there is severe vomiting, the cold capsule will probably not stay down. The generalized allergic reaction can lead to shock and death. Treat the victim for shock and transport it immediately to the veterinarian.

Poisoning

C ats are curious creatures and like to investigate, which leads to many accidental poisonings each year. Often a cat will find an open can or bottle of chemical and, accidentally or on purpose, knock it over. Naturally, the chemical gets on its fur and paws, and while licking the area clean it swallows the possibly toxic substance. It is your responsibility as a pet owner to keep all potentially toxic products tightly closed and out of reach of your cat.

Poisoning symptoms are many and varied, and the toxic substance can be swallowed, absorbed through the skin, or inhaled. Basic emergency treatment for different poisons is as varied as the symptoms, so try to determine the poisoning agent. This is important, because what is correct first aid for one is the wrong treatment for another.

For instance, if the poisoning agent is a corrosive or a petroleum product, you want to forestall vomiting since the returning chemical will cause further irritation and more severe burns. By giving olive oil or egg whites, you are attempting to bind, or tie up, the chemical so that it will not be absorbed.

However, if the chemical is not a corrosive or petroleum product, vomiting should be induced in order to empty the stomach of the poison. Of course, it is unlikely that you will see the poison being swallowed, so in either case, professional help should be sought immediately. If the cat has vomited, the material should be taken with you to the veterinarian for analysis. He will also want you to bring the suspected poison container as this will be of prime importance in determining the most effective treatment.

It is appropriate to mention here the existence of Poison Control Centers located all over the United States and in Canada. On page 6 you'll find space to write the phone number of the center nearest your home. If you ever have a poisoning emergency, they can tell you the appropriate treatment and the proper antidote to give until you get to the veterinarian.

In addition to the obvious poisoning agents, ornamental houseplants can also be dangerous to a cat. It is safe to assume that all common houseplants are toxic to some degree, some more than others.

The best solution is to place the plants in areas where your cat cannot reach them, and use hanging baskets for the more toxic types. If in doubt, call your veterinarian and tell him the type of plant you have or are going to purchase. He will tell you whether or not it poses a hazard.

Fires are another possible threat to cats. Do not risk your own life to save your cat. Leave that task to the firefighters or those trained in rescue. If your cat does suffer from smoke inhalation, get it away from the area and into fresh air. If it is conscious, flush the eyes with diluted boric acid solution or plain water to wash out soot and other particles.

If the animal is not breathing or if the heart is not beating, use artificial respiration and/or CPR. If the smoke is intense, the airway and lungs may also be seriously damaged by inhalation of smoke and heated air. Burned lungs collect fluid, causing shortness of breath. To ease breathing, the cat's head should be kept higher than its body. Also, a burned airway may swell shut; it is imperative to keep this airway open. Immediate professional help is essential.

Carbon monoxide poisoning can be caused by faulty heaters, but it is often due to our own carelessness. Cats often suffer carbon monoxide poisoning from being transported in car trunks. This is dangerous and inhumane.

Characteristic signs are depression, lack of coordination, heavy panting, deep red gums, and possibly convulsions. Oxygen is needed immediately, and the cat should be taken to a veterinarian at once. If there is no heartbeat or respiration, CPR is essential.

Nature provides all life with some means of protection. With certain toads it is the saliva, which is thought to contain a potent toxin.

The poison contained in a toad's saliva is so strong that once it comes in contact with the mouth or eyes of the cat, it causes severe symptoms to develop within minutes. These symptoms include excessive drooling, shaking head and body, lack of coordination, difficulty in breathing, convulsions, and even coma. It affects the heart and nervous system to such a degree that death can occur within 30 minutes if the cat is not treated. It is important to flush the mouth and eyes immediately with copious amounts of water.

In the instance of toad poisoning, start treatment for shock immediately. Immediate veterinary treatment is important in order to save the cat's life.

Puncture Wound

A puncture wound may be difficult to see because it is often covered with hair. The first sign may be a limp if it is on the leg, or slightly blood-tinged fur on other parts of the body.

If the puncture wound is on the body, you can see the extent of the injury more clearly after you have clipped the hair around the area. After cleaning the wound with 3% hydrogen peroxide, examine for an imbedded foreign object, such as a splinter or shard of glass, and remove it if possible. Puncture wounds are deceptive; they can be deeper than they look. These deep wounds often damage muscle tissue, causing fluid to accumulate. It is best to leave the wound open so it can drain. This minimizes the risk of infection and swelling.

An exception to leaving the wound open would be excessive bleeding or a chest wound. Chest wounds can be very serious. If there is a hole through the entire chest wall, a "sucking" noise will be heard as the cat breathes. The act of breathing causes outside air to rush into the chest and around the lungs, causing lung collapse.

Your first priority is to seal the hole quickly to keep air from entering. If a foreign object such as a stick or an arrow is in the chest, do not attempt to pull it out. This could open the hole and lead to lung collapse. Just bandage tightly around the object and take the cat to the veterinarian immediately.

Queening Problems

The beauty of birth is a rewarding experience, but most cats don't want onlookers during delivery. It is important to supply a secluded spot for the queen to have her kittens; yet despite all your preparations, she may have them someplace else.

When you first have reason to believe your cat is pregnant, she should have a prenatal examination by a veterinarian to verify pregnancy and forestall later complications.

The normal length of pregnancy (gestation period) is 63 to 65 days. It is not abnormal to deliver a few days early or late, which presents no cause for alarm as long as the general health of the cat is good. It is a good idea to check with your veterinarian if the cat has not delivered by the 66th day. He or she will examine the cat and make sure that everything is going the way it should. Cats can deliver as late as 70 days and still have normal live kittens.

In preparation for queening, the cat will become very restless and very vocal. Often a queen will dig around the queening box as if nesting, and will lose interest in food. These signs may indicate birth will occur within 24 hours.

The second stage of delivery includes the actual delivery of the kittens which, as has been mentioned, can occur anywhere except where you want it to. When the queen lies on her breastbone with her back legs to the side, you can expect delivery. If a brown or foul-smelling discharge from the vulva is present, contact your veterinarian immediately. When strong contractions begin, the first kitten should be delivered within 30 minutes. Failure to deliver the first kitten after continuous hard labor indicates a problem, and professional help is necessary.

A kitten may be born head first or tail and rear legs first. Both presentations are normal and offer no problems to the queen. Simple directions for assistance in delivery are listed on pages 113-117. You will want to familiarize yourself with these procedures in case they should become necessary.

Some queens will stop labor after the first one or two kittens are born, and not start again for 24 to 48 hours. During this time, they are very calm and nurse the kitten(s) as if there were no more to be delivered. Usually, delivery will start again and normal kittens will be delivered. It is important to be sure the queen is going through this normal stage and not having problems evidenced by depression, lack of appetite, or abnormal discharges from the vulva.

The kittens are delivered in a water-filled sac or membrane. Most queens remove and eat this as soon as the kitten is born. If the mother will not clean the kitten, it is up to you to do it so the kitten can breathe.

After delivery, the queen will be calm as she nurses and cleans her kittens. Don't handle the kittens yourself or allow them to be handled, as this will upset the mother. If there are other animals in the house, they should be kept away. Any attempt to move the kittens away from wherever they were born is futile. The queen will become upset and will return them to their original birthplace.

Shock

Shock is extremely serious—the number one killer in accidents. It is a reaction to heavy internal or external bleeding, or any serious injury that "scares" the body; for example, a large wound or amputation with heavy blood loss.

To compensate for the loss, the heart beats faster; this keeps the blood pressure from falling. The blood vessels that supply the outside of the body narrow. This conserves blood so that vital organs of the body continue to receive their normal blood supply.

However, if there is heavy blood loss or other serious injury, the body overreacts and causes a pooling of blood in the internal organs. This can cause death due to a drop in external blood pressure and possible oxygen starvation of the brain. Pale gums or cold extremities indicate shock.

When shock is present, you want to reverse the process. Elevate the hindquarters to allow more blood to reach the brain. Stop visible bleeding to prevent a drop in blood pressure. Wrap the cat in a blanket with hot water bottles to help keep the body temperature up. This is necessary because the external blood vessels become constricted, and the outside of the body becomes very cold due to lack of normal blood flow. Raising the temperature of the outside of the body helps conserve heat.

Treatment for shock cannot hurt your cat and may save its life. Shock requires professional care, and the victim should be taken to the veterinarian immediately.

Snakebite

Poisonous snakebites are rare in North America. Most snakes are nonpoisonous, and neither poisonous nor nonpoisonous snakes will attack a cat unless provoked. But our pets are curious, and bites will occur.

If you see the cat bitten, try to kill or capture the snake so positive type identification can be made. If this is not possible, try to remember the identifying characteristics of the snake. This will be helpful to your veterinarian.

If you are certain the bite was from a nonpoisonous snake, no danger really exists, except for possible infection from the bite. Since the snake's mouth carries bacteria, clean the wound with 3% hydrogen peroxide and use an antibacterial ointment daily.

If you did not witness the cat being bitten, the diagnosis of snakebite is based on the cat's probable exposure to a snake. Also, note the symptoms that the cat exhibits, listed on pages 125 and 131. Clip the hair around the suspected area to identify the type of bite. Nonpoisonous bites look like fine puncture wounds arranged in a "U" shape. If the bite has two large puncture wounds with several fine puncture wounds behind them, and the area is painful, it is probably poisonous. Immediate treatment will be needed to save the cat's life. If you are not certain that the bite is nonpoisonous, treat it as poisonous.

If the cat is conscious, be sure to restrain it before starting treatment for a poisonous bite. The procedure will definitely be painful.

If the bite is on the leg or tail, it is important to apply a tourniquet because it will slow the spread of the poison throughout the body. Cuts deep enough to draw blood should be made over the fang marks. Then, you must suck the blood from the wound in order to remove as much venom as you can and reduce the amount of poison in the body. Use strong suction and be careful not to swallow the blood. Do not use this technique if you have open sores or cuts on your lips, tongue, or inside cheeks; the poison could be absorbed into your system.

After as much venom as possible has been sucked out, flush thoroughly by pouring 3% hydrogen peroxide into the wound. The application of ice may help to reduce the spread of toxin by constricting blood vessels in the area.

Keep the tourniquet in place while transporting the cat to the veterinarian, loosening it for 10 seconds every 15 minutes, then retightening. If the bite is on the face or body, the same treatment should be followed, but you will not use a tourniquet.

The severity of the reaction caused by any poisonous snakebite will depend on the size of the cat and the closeness of the bite to the